THE
Arthritis
EXERCISE
BOOK

Semyon Krewer
*In collaboration with
Ann Edgar, R.P.T.*

Foreword by
Samuel S. Sverdlik, M.D.

Cornerstone Library
Published by Simon & Schuster
New York

Published by CORNERSTONE LIBRARY
A Simon & Schuster Division of
Gulf & Western Corporation

Simon & Schuster Building
1230 Avenue of the Americas
New York, New York 10020

CORNERSTONE LIBRARY and colophon are trademarks
of Simon & Schuster, registered in the U.S.
Patent and Trademark Office.
Manufactured in the United States of America

Illustrations by Lynn Thompson Welch

10 9 8 7 6 5 4

Library of Congress Cataloging in Publication Data

Krewer, Semyon
    The arthritis exercise book.

    Bibliography: p.
    Includes index.
    1. Arthritis—Prevention. 2. Exercise
therapy. I. Edgar, Ann, joint author. II. Title.
RC933.K73   616.7'22'0624   80-18733

ISBN 0-346-12497-2

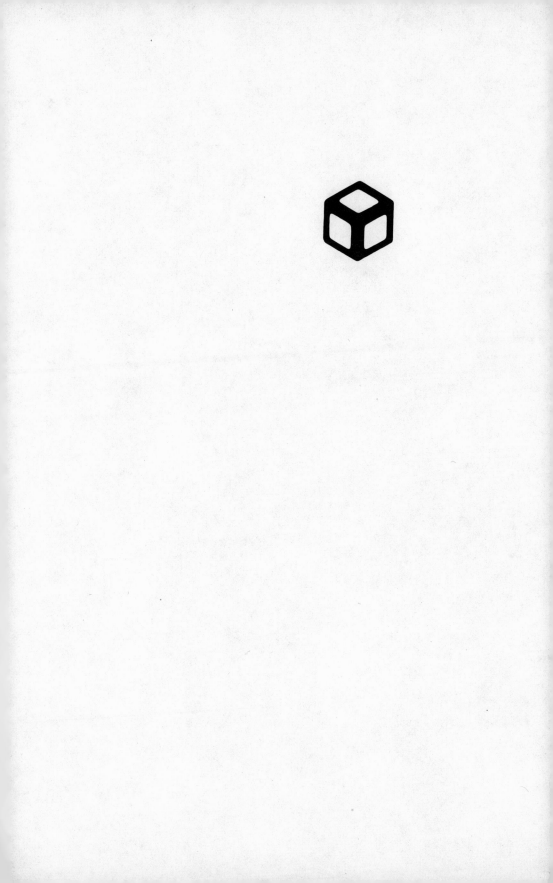

DEDICATED
TO MY WIFE, ELSA, COMRADE IN ARMS
IN MY FIFTEEN-YEAR STRUGGLE
WITH ARTHRITIS

Contents

A Note to the Reader

The exercises in this book are designed to maintain and increase your strength, flexibility, and endurance. They are of special benefit to people over thirty-five years of age, who want to exercise in ways that will protect their joints. The exercises can be considered *preventive*, since they may help to delay the onset of osteoarthritis. If rheumatoid arthritis is present, the exercises can be considered *therapeutic*.

If you are under the care of a physician for the treatment of arthritis, please consult him or her about the exercises that seem best for you.

Important warning: The exercises in this book are not meant to be carried out by persons with severe crippling from rheumatoid arthritis. It would be painful and even harmful for such persons to attempt to stretch themselves to reach the positions described. All exercises in this book are designed to incur practically no pain that would linger for any length of time. If pain should follow any particular exercise, that exercise may not be appropriate for you; consult your physician about it. Your doctor may prescribe a personalized program for you, which may contain some of the exercises in this book.

If you have rheumatoid arthritis, please do not consider exercises and physical therapy exclusive treatment for your condition. These are very important modalities which are only part of an overall medical treatment program consisting of medication, a balanced mix of rest and activity, and physical therapy.

S.K.

Medical Foreword

☐ Osler, in response to a question about living a long life, is said to have answered, "Get a chronic disease and take good care of it."

Semyon Krewer may not have read this admonition, but he has surely followed it. His "owner's manual" for taking good care of his body, particularly those mechanical parts, the muscles, tendons, ligaments, bones, and joints, is truly a comprehensive guide to anyone afflicted with arthritis.

Caring for the mechanical failures in chronic musculoskeletal disorders is the major thrust of this volume. The emphasis is on rest, splints, exercises, and how to use them. There is no panacea, pill, injection, or miracle that can spare the patient who may never have followed a physical conditioning regime previously, and now is advised to do so. This effort requires great discipline. To make the exercise program palatable, it is spread out over a week, a very sensible idea. Dedication to the procedures and careful attention to the suggestions can be invaluable to many readers afflicted with arthritis.

This book is also more than a manual. Its personalized, anecdotal quality speaks to the indomitable will that a man has brought to what could be a crippling disease. This volume's seven-day regimen, side trips, and personal encounters give the readers an insight into the experiences of a remarkable man who has been down a long, twisting, and at times painful road on which many of them are likewise traveling. Mr. Krewer has been there and coped. He shares his experience in a lucid, forthright way. With intelligence, discipline, and commitment he has assembled a guide that will profit anyone suffering from the pangs of arthritis, muscle aches and pains, from the toes to the neck and all parts in between.

In over thirty years of medical practice I have seen many patients who have said, "I guess I have to learn to live with it." My problem has been to teach them how. Mr. Krewer's description of how to live with arthritis and its related disorders should put to rest the conception that "you have to learn to live with it" is the end of the road with no more that can be done. It is actually the beginning of what is the biggest challenge of all—asserting one's will upon one's body to modify and correct the ravages of what could become a serious, disabling disease.

There is always a part a patient can play in the resolution of any illness or disease. People living with disabling diseases must become active partners with their physicians and physicians with their patients in this learning process. A person with arthritis or some related problem must learn all he can about the problem and must mobilize every personal resource toward the goal of properly coping. This is a personal commitment. The physician, therapist, family, and friends all may try to help, but only the individual himself can achieve the goals—each in time.

Of course, to "live with" is not to conquer. Having arthritis, particularly rheumatoid arthritis, is not a game you are out to win. Neither should it become one you must lose. The latter is really not the attitude to take as either a patient, physician, or therapist. The goal is to *cope*, and to cope intelligently is to learn all you can about the disease. As a practitioner of Rehabilitation Medicine for many years, I find that there is much to learn in this volume. It will now be a companion to me, to many of my staff, and above all to patients and their families.

It is a tour de force in the genre of how-to books and should be as valuable to physicians, therapists, and families as it is to patients.

SAMUEL S. SVERDLIK, M.D.
Director, Department of Rehabilitation Medicine
St. Vincent's Hospital and Medical Center
New York City

Clinical Professor of Rehabilitation Medicine
New York University College of Medicine

Acknowledgments

□ Some years ago I became involved in the Student Help for the Elderly program at Columbia University, first as one of those benefiting from the help provided by the program, and later as a member of the Board of Student Help. It seemed to me that the program could be more effective if the students were better informed about suitable exercises for the elderly, especially those with arthritis. My suggestion to this effect was well received, but we could not at that time find any literature that furnished detailed instructions.

The local chapter of the Arthritis Foundation referred us to Ann Edgar, R.P.T., a graduate in physical therapy from the faculty of medicine, Columbia University, who instructed some of the students in assisting in home exercise programs. I saw then the need for a book combining detailed, well-illustrated exercise instructions—especially for isometric exercises, which are frequently recommended but almost nowhere properly described. This book, I hope, will answer that need. My aim has been to update the range-of-motion exercises familiar to many arthritics and to introduce the modern, well-proven hold-relax technique of proprioceptive neuromuscular facilitation (PNF) into the home exercise program. Whereas in the hold-relax technique, the patient has to strain against the resisting hand of the therapist. Miss Edgar taught me that once you learn body awareness you can tense muscles without external resistance. It is well documented that muscle relaxation follows muscle tension, whether against external resistance or not. This fact permits the use of the method I call the "tense-relax-and-stretch" technique to be carried out at home without the aid of a helper.

Miss Edgar was instrumental in helping to refine this technique during our many sessions over a period of several years. She helped to determine just where this technique works best and where gentle range-of-motion exercises are more appropriate.

One of the important aspects of the hold-relax technique is that it is more pain-free, more effective, and less time-consuming than the older exercises in which the limbs are moved repeatedly and sometimes painfully through the full range of motion.

I owe a debt of gratitude also to Dr. Edward Lowman, Clinical Director of the Institute of Rehabilitation Medicine, New York University Medical Center, for sponsoring a clinical evaluation of the Hand Gym, which I designed for my own use. One outcome of the study was a set of detailed instructions for using the Hand Gym, prepared by the occupational therapy department of the Institute. Dr. Lowman facilitated my carrying out myographic research (measurement of electrical impulses accompanying muscle contractions), which enabled me to design isometric exercises for the Hand Gym.

I wish to thank Dr. Samuel Sverdlik, director of the rehabilitation medicine department at St. Vincent's Hospital, New York City, for supervising a clinical study of twenty-three arthritic patients using the Hand Gym, that included a four-year follow-up. This work convinced me that a well-illustrated exercise system could be carried out effectively at home.

I am grateful to Dr. Valery Lanyi of the arthritis clinic at Bellevue Hospital, New York City, for encouraging me to pursue my analysis of the interconnection of lymphatic function, arthritic symptoms, and modalities of physical therapy.

In designing the exercises, I had in mind also the words of caution I have heard from many rheumatologists, notably Dr. George Ehrlich of the Albert Einstein Hospital in Philadelphia, about the current popularity of jogging and tennis. Persons who are prone to osteoarthritis may hasten the onset of this condition by engaging in sports of this sort, which place severe stress on the weight-bearing joints. A recent survey by the National Cancer Institute indicated that increased longevity may be expected as people exercise more and eat more prudently, but early osteoarthritis should not be the penalty for exercise. By following the exercise system in this book, people of middle age and up should be able to maintain or increase their flexibility, strength, and endurance without damaging their joints.

For help in analyzing certain aspects of physiology and anatomy, I am grateful to my daughter, Julie Ann Krewer.

I thank my friend Charles C. Bennett for helping me to present new ideas in physical therapy for arthritics to the profession and—once these approaches were found to be beneficial—for helping me to make this information more widely available to the public.

Finally, I wish to acknowledge the careful work of Lynn Thompson Welch in preparing the numerous illustrations for this book, which promote body awareness by their remarkable sense of body movement.

SEMYON KREWER
Point Lookout, New York

Introduction: Wake Up Your Sense of Well-Being

☐ Remember childhood? You liked your body then. Probably like other children you flexed your biceps for admiring relatives, felt pride as your height increased, looked in the mirror at your developing self with feelings of wonderment and anticipation. You seemed to have endless energy for your games and activities, and the more active you were, the happier you felt. What you may not realize is that the child you once were—the child who so enjoyed play and movement—is still very much a part of you.

As human beings, we are by nature constructed to move about—at times vigorously and strenuously. Primitive people had to move about most of their waking hours in search of food and shelter. But beyond the activity that is necessary to sustain life, movement has always been enjoyed for its own sake. People of all cultures throughout history have deliberately moved their bodies in dance, sport, and other exercise, and have celebrated the active body in books, music, sculpture, and other arts (figs. 1 and 2). We all respond to physical performance, either as spectators or as performers ourselves. Very recent times have seen a surge of participation in various forms of physical exercise. Joggers populate the pathways of our parks and streets. Dance and exercise groups spring into being

1. *David, by Michelangelo:*
strength and beauty

2. *Ballerina:*
flexibility and elegance

all around us. Skiing, water sports, and a variety of racquet games are gaining enthusiasts in all age groups.

More and more of us are discovering the necessity for deliberate exercising. We must have bodily movement to maintain strength, endurance, and flexibility. Through exercise we can carry the load of our daily work without fatigue. *Heightened well-being induced by exercise gives us an improved mental and emotional state.*

Our need for purposeful exercise is enhanced by the pushbutton age in which we live. Especially after age forty, we are likely to find the physical demands of our work and home life greatly reduced. Many labor-saving devices and the ever-present automobile for use on short errands as well as longer trips all contribute to our becoming unhealthily sedentary. Lately, the threat of overweight, lowered well-being, and cardio-vascular disease has prodded thousands of people to take up the sport of running.

But there are many—including the estimated forty million who suffer from arthritis—for whom exercise is just as vitally important, but who may injure themselves with activities that place excessive stress on the joints, particularly on the ankles, knees, and hips. What can the arthritic person do to achieve the well-being that exercise provides, without endangering the joints?

WHY WE HAVE TO EXERCISE

☐ For arthritics and all other people, life processes require physical movement. The lymphatic circulation, an intricate drainage system that helps to take wastes and infection out of the body, keeps moving with the aid of bodily movements—the squeezing effect of muscles. Muscles, blood, and bone all require body action. When a broken bone immobilizes an arm or a leg, the forced inactivity during healing allows bone stuff to wash away, and causes that bone to become more porous, weaker than its mate. When motion is resumed, the bone puts down new material and grows stronger again. Prolonged illness in bed brings on wasting of muscles, which regain their size and strength only when regular exercising begins again.

Hospital patients who cannot move themselves are exercised in bed by assistants, for fear the blood will pool in the legs and set loose in the blood vessels a thrombus, or clot, which may fatally strike the lungs, heart, or brain. Many of our movements—stretching, yawning, turning over in bed—are involuntary responses to the physical urge for action.

FUNCTIONING AT YOUR BEST

☐ We cannot stress too much the need for arthritics to religiously follow an exercise program to keep up the functioning of their limbs and to delay disability. Once a disability or deformity has occurred, undoing the damage is extremely difficult; the challenge is that much greater. Regarding my present hip condition, an orthopedic surgeon told me after viewing my X-rays, "I don't understand how you can walk at all." But I did walk, although not very rapidly, thanks to the help I got from well-exercised leg and hip muscles.

In this book, I describe a wide selection of exercises designed to increase range of motion and strength and to improve general health without injuring joints that may already be compromised by arthritis or some other potentially disabling condition. These exercises are both *prophylactic* (preventive) and *therapeutic* (aimed at remedying existing problems), and are designed to help those who are threatened by or who already have painful or restricting conditions. I intend this book to be helpful for all people past age thirty-five, a milestone in life after which osteoarthritis often manifests itself. I hope it will be read by those who are younger and who want to protect their joints, and particularly by those who are determined, as I am, to avoid becoming dependent on others and to function despite severe conditions such as rheumatoid arthritis.

It has been my observation that people battling a disabling disease too often turn to exercise as a last resort, after trying pain medications, muscle relaxants, and even surgery. (And even after surgery, you must exercise to get the skeletal muscles working again.) And, unfortunately, arthritis exercises are seldom presented in a nonpunishing, nonmedical way; usually they are handed down as something to be "complied with."

FINDING THE RIGHT MOTIVATION

☐ Relaxation and body awareness are fundamental to the system of exercise described in these pages. Both techniques are becoming extremely popular today. They are taught and used in classes, group activities, and even clinical treatment. In body-awareness classes, members are asked to touch the various joints of the body and to observe them in action. People learning relaxation techniques are asked to contract and relax in sequence the various muscles and muscle groups and to observe—and feel—the effects. I agree wholeheartedly with the wisdom of this approach. I think that any exercise system that does not explain the reasons why, that does not fully acquaint you with your body, is doomed to fail.

Everything in this book has been tested by my own experiences and learning. I am now, after fifteen years as an arthritic, still reasonably ambulatory and adept with my hands. I do not recommend this system of exercise for arthritics who are severely crippled, however; my experience does not correspond to that condition. People who are severely handicapped will, I hope, be getting treatment and guidance in the management of their disease from physicians and therapists. On the other hand, early arthritics, including those who are not yet fully diagnosed, should become aware of what physical therapy and exercise can do for them. Such programs, I have found, are neglected as part of the total care approach; if begun early, they could prevent a lot of discomfort and crippling.

THE DAILY FIVE-MINUTE TENSE-RELAX-AND-STRETCH EXERCISES

☐ The last chapter of this book details a daily five-minute preventive exercise session. Although it comes at the back of the book (for ready reference), it is the heart and soul of this system of exercise for arthritis. To succeed in maintaining function and combatting pain, resolve to spend those five minutes every day performing the exercises. Then, carry through on the resolution.

After you have read the main part of the book, which details exercises for every part of the body and the reasons why they are effective, it will be clear to you that the daily five-minute session is designed to achieve maximum efficiency in a very brief span of time. I hope you will be eager to achieve what is so readily within reach.

You need not read this book in chapter sequence. Select a topic and browse in it. If you want, skip anything that looks at first like heavy reading. You can come back to these parts later or omit them altogether. My aim has been to make all chapters stand on their own, so that you can read any chapter without having to refer to any other.

In addition to the daily five-minute session in the morning, I strongly advocate a weekly regimen of six five-to-fifteen-minute sessions before bedtime, to be worked out according to your own particular needs. Choose one exercise set for each week night. Your regimen might be as follows:

Monday night:	Neck and jaw—five minutes
Tuesday night:	Shoulders and elbows—ten minutes
Wednesday night:	Hands and wrists—five–ten minutes
Thursday night:	Posture and upper back—five–ten minutes
Friday night:	Hips, lower back, and knees—fifteen minutes
Saturday night:	Feet and ankles—five minutes

In addition, any range of motion that gives you trouble should be practiced at least once daily, regardless of the category.

Do not consider this book a substitute for seeing a physical therapist, if you are able to see one. In addition to teaching you exercises, it is meant to make you more knowledgeable about your body and about physical therapy so that you will be able to converse more accurately with your physician. The more knowledgeable you are, the more fruitful the relationship with your physician will be. Many times a harried physician has used a vocabulary unfamiliar to patients. That is why, in this book, I try to familiarize you with this vocabulary concerning joints and muscles. Once you learn it, it takes you less time to communicate. If you do see a physical therapist, that person should evaluate your ranges of motion, train you in carrying out exercises, and encourage you to do them daily. I have heard a lot about "compliance" in connection with exercises. I think the motivation should come out of your own awareness and not from expected punishment or praise by your therapist.

After many years with arthritis, I have found that the best way to strike back at this disease is to exercise regularly. But, in advocating exercise, I add these important cautions:

1. Do not overexercise.
2. Do not neglect your medical routine.
3. Follow rest schedules.
4. Never exercise until painful unless under the advice of physician.

Part 1

INCLUDES: HOW
the body functions, the rationale for the exercises,
some details about the arthritic disease process, and a
discussion of pain and how to deal with it.

All this information helps to provide a motivation
and a basis for carrying out the exercises in part 2. You
do not have to read all of part 1 in order to do the
exercises in part 2. Each chapter stands on its own and
does not require reading of any other chapter of the
book.

I suggest that you scan the topics in part 1 and
browse in them from time to time; return to any relevant chapter when you need it. The sooner you get to
the exercises in part 2, the better.

THE CHAPTERS

Mobilizing to Fight Arthritis 1

☐ Here, in part 1, I want to prepare my readers for the total body exercise system that follows in part 2 and, in addition, to discuss a well-rounded program for managing arthritis and for living productively despite the presence of the disease. From joint protection, to splints and other devices, to the possible benefits of visiting a spa—this information will, I hope, give arthritics the kind of practical morale-boosting guidance we all look for and need.

MY EXPERIENCE WITH ARTHRITIS

☐ Although I was in treatment from the start with my rheumatoid arthritis, it was four years before I began working with a physical therapist, and then only because I had developed a hand exercise program (described later) that was of interest to the profession. True, my rheumatologist gave me various sheets with descriptions of exercises (lacking illustrations) which I was supposed to perform faithfully. I found these descriptions too abbreviated; the reasons for doing them were not made clear. Morever, they were simply too strenuous to carry out.

After about ten years of the disease I was placed in

a hospital to "regain strength" and improve my flexibility. At the end of the hospital stay I was taught some exercises for home use, and I subsequently studied for myself the biomechanical and physiological rationale of these exercises. I wanted to find the most pain-free way to do them, since pain discourages the performance of any exercise. The most dramatic test of the efficiency of exercise came when I developed a serious arthritic hip condition. Once a week for three months I worked with a therapist on stretching and strengthening the muscles of the hip. Again I confirmed what I had found out earlier in connection with the fingers, neck, knees, ankles, feet, and jaw. Exercises do help to improve function. Thanks to the therapy the pain was lessened and I maintained and even somewhat improved my limited ability to walk.

The exercises I describe incorporate techniques such as isometrics and PNF (proprioceptive neuromuscular facilitation), which increase their efficiency and allow them to be done in less time, with less strain, and with a lower expenditure of energy than in older methods. The system stresses self-help, but it also shows how you can benefit from working with another person—a therapist or understanding helper.

CHECKPOINTS IN THE PROGRESS OF RHEUMATOID ARTHRITIS

☐ To help you judge when and how to exercise I will present here a very abridged description of the timetables in the disease process and the corresponding disabilities. If you are in treatment, your physician and your therapist will direct you in this matter. The material I am presenting may help you to understand their advice.

As you may know, the progression of rheumatoid arthritis is episodic. The episodes may be as short as a week, or they may go on for a long time. I have suffered episodes lasting more than a year. During an episode you can consider that the disease is *active*. At the end of the episode, the disease becomes inactive and you speak of a *remission*. In some cases the patient may suffer only one single episode, and no second or future episodes occur. But often the disease flares up again. After a second or third episode, it may then terminate in a remission. If the flare-ups continue over a period of years, the disease finally reaches a chronic stage in which inflammation may or may not be present, but joints have suffered a lot of destruction, and contractures and deformities have set in, possibly to the point where intensive rehabilitation or reconstructive surgery are called for. (In my case, the inflammatory process, which is specific for rheumatoid arthritis, was eventually suppressed through gold treatment (monthly injections of a gold solution called Myochrysine).

Typically, during the active phase, I found that one or a few joints, usually the knuckles, became inflamed for limited periods of time, and then the inflammation (redness, heat, and swelling) shifted to other joints. Morning stiffness did not last very long, perhaps less than an hour. Fever was not present, and fatigue was not so great as to prevent near-normal activity.

At some point during the active phase, the subacute condition develops into an acute condition. Now the joints become strongly inflamed and the inflammation does not disappear in a few days; fever may be present, and morning stiffness lasts for several hours. Activity is greatly reduced due to fatigue. Although there is variation from one patient to another, the acute phase should not last longer than one or, at most, two weeks if your joints are given a complete rest. Sometimes hospitalization is recommended in severe cases. Usually in this period, a variety of anti-inflammatory drugs are given to reduce the joint inflammation and thus help bring the acute phase to an end. This is a dangerous time during which much joint destruction is liable to take place. Joints are supposed to be rested completely during this time. Therefore, *no active motion exercises should be done.* Isometric exercises are permitted. However, to avoid the danger of adhesions developing near the joint, which would affect elements of the joint such as muscle and capsule tissue and produce severe limitations of joint movement, each joint should be moved passively through the complete range of motion once a day. As the acute phase nears an end, which becomes evident through the fact that all symptoms are lessening, the patient is usually encouraged to do active range-of-motion exercises. The physician makes the important judgment on when to resume a full program of exercises.

In other words, exercises are indicated during all phases of rheumatoid arthritis, except that during the acute phase motion exercises are passive; that is, they are administered by a therapist or helper to maintain range of motion. The choice of exercises and the overall amount should be discussed with your physician. I describe in this book exercises that are designed to be as pain-free as possible. *If you encounter any pain at all, discuss this with your physician or therapist. Don't try to tough it out.*

OSTEOARTHRITIS

☐ Osteoarthritis is called the noninflammatory arthritis, although a small amount of heat can be detected on damaged joints, which is indicative of inflammation. (I experienced this with my knees, where a localized area felt warm when I placed my palm over it.) Osteoarthritis is a slowly progressing disease in which the cartilage covering the ends of bones that form the joints is used up and not replaced. One discriminates between *primary* and *secondary* osteoarthritis. Primary osteoarthritis occurs with progressing age. It can start as early as age forty, but the majority of cases seems to occur after age sixty. As the cartilage is depleted, and the joint space thereby reduced, the joint becomes less efficient in function. At first it is uncomfortable and finally it becomes painful. Secondary osteoarthritis is induced either by repetitive trauma (dressmakers and typists can develop arthritic fingers) or by a single trauma to a joint (one patient caught her fingers in a garage door and developed osteoarthritis thereafter). Osteoarthritis resulting from sport injuries may occur at any age. Remember that at age thirty-five you are more prone to slight injuries than at twenty.

The medications most helpful in osteoarthritis are painkillers like aspirin or Tylenol, although the anti-inflammatory action of some drugs like Indocin and Clinoril may also be helpful.

WHERE TO SEEK TREATMENT

☐ Of course, the first move to make when arthritis strikes is to seek sound medical advice. What can we expect from physicians and therapists? In most illnesses, we usually turn to our *general practitioner* or *internist* for relief. He or she is most familiar with our lifestyle and medical history and can usually *diagnose* the condition and prescribe the proper treatment. If the treatment does not succeed as expected, we may be sent to consult with a specialist, a *rheumatologist,* who is trained to establish the diagnosis, that is, to tell us which type of arthritis we have, if any. Diagnosis can be a very complex procedure, requiring many blood tests, X-rays, physical evaluation, and so on. The rheumatologist evaluates these tests and prescribes the proper treatment.

If you have osteoarthritis, most probably you won't need continued treatment by a rheumatologist. He usually reports back to the general practitioner with the diagnosis and recommendation for treatment, which will probably include pain-relieving medication and exercises, as well as other physical therapy modalities.

In the case of *gout,* another form of arthritis, you will probably come under the definite regimen of medication and diet which helps this condition considerably; it can usually be supervised adequately by the general practitioner.

Arthritis caused by infection may be treated with antibiotics and often completely cured. This was the experience of a relative of mine who developed a serious inflammation of her osteoarthritic knees, due to hepatitis. The symptoms disappeared when the hepatitis was overcome.

There are many additional conditions, some of which are highly complex, which can produce arthritic symptoms. One of these is the disease *lupus erythematosus,* which requires close supervision by a specialist. In my case, many tests were performed before lupus could be eliminated as the cause of my arthritic complaints.

Psoriasis is often accompanied by arthritic symptoms. I have seen finger joints and knees involved due to psoriasis.

Establishing the diagnosis of rheumatoid arthritis may take time. When my medical diagnosis was finally established, it was two years after the onset of the disease. When I expressed my happiness to my rheumatologist, he was very surprised. "What are you so happy about?" he asked. I answered, "Now that we know what it is, we can fight it." He grinned and replied, "You have a rocky road ahead!" And he was right. We both would have preferred one of the types of arthritis that has a clear-cut, definitive treatment method and can be expected to subside. But I am an optimist by nature, and have faithfully followed all the recommendations of my doctor—even those that tested my resourcefulness, like having to use splints. It was something of a research project finding a hospital where they could be made.

If you want to inform yourself fully about the many types of arthritis, you can request literature from the *Arthritis Foundation*. And there are quite a few fine books written by physicians on the subject.

My point is that *it is extremely important to establish a correct diagnosis of the type of arthritis present*. Only then can you and your doctors chart the proper course of action.

The *physiatrist* is a physician who specializes in physical medicine and rehabilitation, and who knows a great deal about kinesiology and exercise. We may be referred to him by the general practitioner, internist, or rheumatologist. He is experienced in understanding the various sources of pain and deformity, and in choosing the treatment modalities that will be most helpful in alleviating pain and improving our functioning. The array of techniques includes exercise, heat in various applications (hot packs, ultrasound), transcutaneous nerve stimulation (TNS), deep relaxation, and possibly acupuncture, at the chronic stage.

Your physiatrist may assign you to a *physical therapist* or an *occupational therapist,* or both. He also may prescribe various forms of treatment. In the early years of arthritis, these professionals are supposed to help you set up your home maintenance program if you are not able to do this by yourself. After later follow-ups, the physiatrist may prescribe splints for individual joints; these will be individually fitted by an occupational or physical therapist.

In the later years of arthritis, the physical therapist administers therapeutic exercise several times a week to correct deformities, and may also administer hot packs and ultrasound treatment, and help you in fitting any canes or walkers that may be necessary. The occupational therapist, in later years, may advise you of how to select a wheelchair and suggest adaptive devices for the bathroom and the kitchen that are designed to make daily living easier.

THE RHEUMATOLOGIST'S SPECIAL ROLE

☐ You may ask, "What remains for the rheumatologist to do?" Plenty. Apart from being in charge of your pharmaceutical regimen, which is a balancing act between drugs and their side effects, he or she will perform general medical checkups to observe your total health picture. Rheumatoid arthritis can attack, directly or indirectly, any organ of the body—directly, by invading organs with the disease; indirectly, through the various side effects of medications (for example, aspirin on the stomach, and cortisone on both the stomach and heart). The rheumatologist checks also whether any pains in the body are coming from diseases other than arthritis. After all, cancer also produces nagging, consistent pain. The rheumatologist also tries to consult with you on a balanced lifestyle and the work you can do within the limits of your joint range, just as a doctor advises a cardiac patient to live within the limits of his heart capacity. Thus, the responsibility of the rheumatologist is great.

I have found all the physicians who have ever helped me with my arthritis to be very concerned people. They have tried to give me the benefit of their experience with the many, many patients they have observed. It has been said of arthritis that no two cases are alike. The severity of the disease and the length of time the disease lasts are different for all arthritics. It follows, then, that physicians may vary widely in their opinions. Do not expect a consensus on what is the best treatment schedule. Rely on your rheumatologist, or—if you are a patient at an arthritis clinic where you are seen by various physicians—rely on the consensus they form about your case. Don't be upset by a divergence of medical opinion. Remember that you, as the patient, are the only real judge of whether you are doing better. This so-called self-assessment is a very important feedback for the physician or the clinic staff with whom you will chart your future course.

Rheumatoid arthritis, as I have said, is a disease of ups and downs, of flare-ups and remissions. Some lucky people have only one or two flare-ups followed by complete remission. Most of us, however, continue with the ups and downs. We have remissions between flare-ups, but the remissions are not complete; with each flare-up the joints are further damaged, muscles are weakened, and function is reduced.

The level of disease activity during the subacute period may be different for different patients. My rheumatologist described my case as a continuous, smoldering process, with tissue destruction continuing at a slow rate. Now, in the chronic stage, I am mainly concerned with keeping my body as fit as possible and not succumbing to inertia, which undoubtedly would make me an invalid.

SEEK OUT THE RIGHT HELP

☐ We have to remain optimistic. For all of us, at every stage of the disease, something medical and physical can be done to help. It is up to us, however, to scramble for the right help. We cannot expect from any individual physician to get all the information or provide all the help possible. Medicine is a very, very wide field, and no physician can be expected to know and be able to carry out all the possible procedures. But our chief attending physician should be able to refer us to the appropriate specialists—to the orthopedic surgeon, or physiatrist, or physical or occupational therapist whose particular skills can help us. The Arthritis Foundation supplies names of physicians who specialize in treatment of arthritic patients. These are mostly rheumatologists, but in some regions the lists also contain names of general practitioners, orthopedic surgeons, and physiatrists. The Arthritis Foundation can also furnish the names of rehabilitation institutions, arthritis clinics, and occupational and physical therapy departments of hospitals in your area. To obtain outpatient treatment in these places, referral by your personal physician usually is required.

THE LESS STRESS THE BETTER

☐ Physicians are agreed that it is particularly important for arthritics to keep in good health, to avoid colds as much as possible, and to reduce the stresses of life. The general reserve of strength in rheumatoid arthritics is so reduced that any additional strain or stress takes a disproportionate toll. We may have to accept, either by choice or necessity, a cutback on our own normal level of work. Trying to do our accustomed work in spite of reduced strength may provoke a flare-up.

The stresses to be avoided include mental or emotional stresses, which are known to be a contributing factor to the onset of arthritis as well as to the occurrence of flare-ups. I was told by one physician in charge of a hospital ward for rheumatoid arthritics that on Mondays, following the excitement of Sunday visits by relatives, many patients felt worse.

There are direct stresses on the body, such as the climatic stress of cold or humid weather. A drop in barometric pressure seems especially stressful for arthritics. To counteract such stresses, we try to wear appropriate clothing and keep our homes comfortable and free of drafts. Some people even spend winters in the sun belt to remain in a favorable climate throughout the year.

Another type of stress on the body is the lack of proper nutrition, which can result in poor bowel functions and symptoms of iron and vitamin deficiency.

THE KEY IS PROPHYLAXIS

□ Although we cannot cure our arthritis, where stress is concerned there is much that we can do to help ourselves. Here I come to that large field which is called "prophylaxis" in rheumatoid arthritis and which is largely the subject of this book. Exercise is one of the most helpful and least utilized techniques of prophylaxis.

I knew little about arthritis in my younger days, but an accident that occurred to a close relative taught me something about osteoarthritis. While playing a game at school she injured her kneecaps, which then started to deteriorate. Her experience demonstrated how a joint that is eroded and not well aligned becomes susceptible to colds, hepatitis, and other ills. Once I contracted rheumatoid arthritis, I realized that I must be kind to my joints, keep them free of stress, and prevent, if possible, infections that might settle in them. This is the first step in the process of "babying oneself." It is one of the main prophylactic measures we can use to help deflect the course of the disease.

I have learned, furthermore, that one can relieve the inflammation of the joints through complete rest. I now understand the reason for this after experiencing the use of the hand-rest splints. I found that wearing hand-rest splints throughout the night helped considerably to reduce the swelling of my finger joints. If hand-rest splints are not worn during the night the assumption would be that one's hands would still be rested, but apparently the degree of rest they receive is not sufficient; the slightest movement of the hands and fingers during sleep seems to impede the process of reducing inflammation. Similarly for larger joints, you get more benefit from resting comfortably in bed, with a minimum of tossing and turning, than from sitting in a chair and moving only slightly.

Another prophylactic measure is to use an inflamed joint only as much as you can without aggravating it. Let me give you an example. My finger joints were quickly rid of inflammation and made painless by cortisone injections. But after I wrote two pages in longhand, the inflammation recurred and I had to see my rheumatologist for another injection. The lesson to be learned from this is that we have to find the level at which we can use our joints and function, but not use them so much that we aggravate their condition and bring on inflammation. The judgment can come only from your personal observation, because the degree of one's susceptibility to inflammation is directly related to the severity of the disease, and this changes from time to time.

We can expect our physicians to prescribe all possible inflammation-reducing and disease-suppressing drugs, but we can also help ourselves by using the prophylactic means that are available to reduce inflammation. And, most important, we can strive to keep our limbs and body flexible and the muscles as strong and efficient as possible, so as to prevent crippling and loss of function. For most of us, the chances of succeeding in this are excellent. I have found that determination and insight are necessary if we are to do the required exercises and to use the other modalities.

There is always a danger that someone reading about the conditions of serious arthritis will become alarmed and discouraged. That is why I like to put the emphasis on prophylaxis—changes in lifestyle, prudence in expending one's energy, daily exercise (very brief sessions), and developing an understanding of how the body works so that we can make intelligent use of splints and other devices and monitor our bodily functions.

THE STRATEGY FOR FATIGUE

□ From the onset of my arthritis, I was not able to give more than two hours at a time to any of my normal activities without becoming so fatigued that I had to rest. I found out through experience that total, complete rest, preferable in bed, for an hour or two, resulted in more energy for my next back-to-work session of two hours. Sitting in a chair, perhaps reading a book, is *not* a complete rest.

It is remarkable how relatively little effort is needed to take care of our daily needs, compared with the strength we normally exert as healthy people. One-third to one-quarter of the normal strength seems quite all right for me, as long as I retain flexibility. I have learned, however, that in order to maintain even this reduced strength, I require a once-a-week isometric strengthening workout of my muscles; it takes only a few minutes a day for various muscle groups, if spread out over a whole week.

Obviously we want to take the least amount of time out of our day for rehabilitation—for exercise, hot packs, and so forth. This is what this book is all about. If you allot five to ten minutes in the morning plus a short period in the evening to do exercises that are not overly strenuous, you give yourself the best chance of being able to continue your normal, useful activities.

BALANCING REST AND ACTIVITY

□ Judging the proper mix of rest and activity is crucial. I would like to illuminate this matter in a basic way so that you will be able to figure out, at any one time, whether to rest or to be active.

If we remain in bed for several days, our joints will become less inflamed. If we then get up and are active for a very short time, without aggravating the joints, and then return to bed, there is a chance that the disease process will remain well under control. Such a program is unrealistic, however: first, because we would become too weak, the muscles would get flabby; second, because inactivity is distressing and makes daily life seem less worthwhile. So we have to be active as long as we can.

I suggest this formula for a proper mix of rest and activity:

1. Allot the necessary time for exercise so that the body will be sufficiently strong and flexible to maintain activity.
2. Allow for time in bed—sleeping and resting with the least possible aggravation of the joints.
3. Use the remaining time for the activities of daily living: household chores, work, entertainment.

This means that we have to experiment and discover for ourselves how much time we can sneak away for the fruitful activities that make life useful and happy.

Body Mechanics 2

☐ If the human body came with an owner's manual, complete with parts list and repair hints, many of our health problems could be solved easily. But this is not the case. The body is a mystery to most of us, despite what we learn about it in health and biology classes at school. Not even a physician can be expected to know everything about the body, its malfunctioning, and its repair. That is why there are so many specialists in medicine who concern themselves with a limited aspect of the body.

If we have arthritis, it is important to increase our knowledge of the body. We are concerned with the whole body, not only the skeleton and the muscles and ligaments, but also the temperature, circulation, breathing, and some aspects of the nervous system. Increased knowledge will help us to observe our condition and describe it to our physician and, most importantly, will enable us to understand the reasons for the prophylactic measures that are recommended to us, especially exercises.

OUR MARVELOUS BODY RESOURCES

☐ Essentially the human is an animal that moves about and adapts itself to needs. When the body is not sufficiently used, it loses the capacity to make the most of its possibilities. Bones and teeth decalcify if not used, muscles become flabby and weak when they are not regularly exercised. On the other hand, if demand on the body increases, we have a remarkable capacity to adapt ourselves to the demands. When called upon to function, muscles can increase in bulk, and bones and ligaments can become stronger.

The body also can adapt itself to hot and cold climates, to high and low humidity, and to varying air pressure. The healthy body, furthermore, has a remarkable capacity for self-repair. A cut in the skin will heal by itself, and a broken bone, when properly set, will become as strong as before.

Both adaptability and self-repair are somewhat limited in arthritics. They can never develop the muscle bulk of the "bodybuilder," for instance, since their damaged joints prevent the muscles from being exercised to their limit. In arthritis, also, there is a lessening of adaptability to climatic changes, especially to cold, humidity, and changes in air pressure. As far as self-repair is concerned, it no longer holds true for the joint structures. Cartilage, once used up, is not replaced. Ligaments, once stretched, do not regain their original elasticity.

Arthritics, then, have to follow a narrow, prophylactic path. We have to avoid excesses to which we cannot adapt ourselves. We have to prevent as much damage as possible in order to reduce the need for repair.

THE EXERCISER'S VOCABULARY

☐ I will start the discussion of the human body with a review of the skeleton (fig. 1) and of some of the nomenclature of interest to arthritics, including words used in anatomy to describe directions and locations of certain parts of the body. This will help you to converse better with your physician or therapist.

Anterior denotes everything located on the front part of the body; *posterior* anything on the back of the body. Moving the extremities laterally (to the side, away from the center line of the body) is *abduction*. Moving the extremities medially (toward the center line of the body) is *adduction*.

When referring to hands, abduction and adduction respectively mean moving the fingers away from the

1. *Front (anterior) view of skeleton*

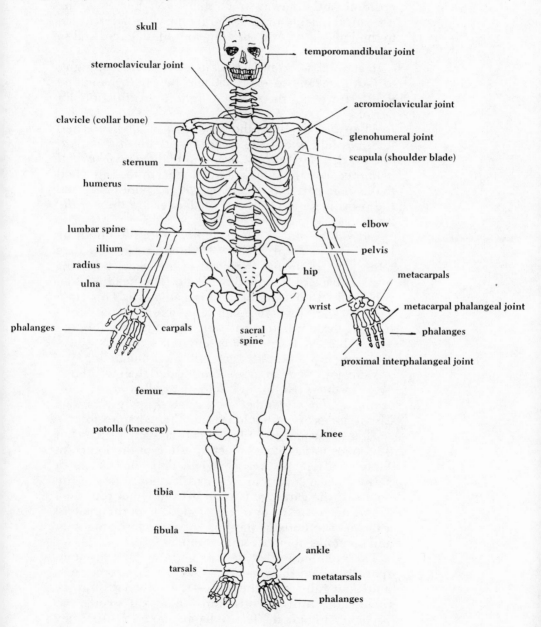

skull — temporomandibular joint

sternoclavicular joint

acromioclavicular joint

clavicle (collar bone) — glenohumeral joint

sternum — scapula (shoulder blade)

humerus

lumbar spine — elbow

illium — pelvis

radius — hip

ulna

wrist — metacarpals

metacarpal phalangeal joint

phalanges — carpals — sacral spine — phalanges

proximal interphalangeal joint

femur

patolla (kneecap) — knee

tibia

fibula

ankle

tarsals — metatarsals

phalanges

middle line (the middle finger) and moving them toward the middle line.

The word *proximal* (in proximity) means a position closer to the body; the word *distal* (more distant), a position farther away from the body. For example, note on the skeleton that the femur bone is proximal to the knee joint, and the tibia and fibula are distal to the knee joint.

In general, to *extend* a joint means to hold it straight; to *flex* it means to exert muscle power to bend the joint. However, there is no definitive direction for *flexion*.

When we talk about the *phalanges* of the hands and feet, we talk about the fingertips as the *distal phalanges;* they are farthest from the body. The *proximal phalanges* are the bones of the fingers or toes attached to the main part of the hand or foot; the bones between the proximal and the distal phalanges are the *middle phalanges.*

Individual bones form *joints* with neighboring bones. These joints, most of which are flexible, are often formed so that the head of the distal bone fits into the base of the proximal bone. The head is often spherical and fits the base of the adjoining bone in a way that permits both bones to rotate in several directions. An example of a ball-and-socket joint is the hip. The spherical head of the femur fits into its corresponding firm base, the acetabulum, in the pelvis.

Many joints are far more complicated than this, however. In the wrist, for example, the radius of the forearm *articulates* (contacts and rotates) against various carpal bones. The shoulder is another complex joint.

There is usually a lining of cartilage on the ends of the bones to facilitate smooth gliding of the joint. An X-ray of a joint shows what is called joint space—a narrow space separating the cartilaginous ends of the bones. If the cartilage is used up and is not replaced, as in osteoarthritis, or if it is eroded, as in rheumatoid arthritis, the ends of the bones come closer together and one talks about a reduced joint space.

The membrane that defines and encloses the joint space is called the *synovium* (see fig. 2); it secretes a fluid that lubricates the joint—the synovial fluid. In rheumatoid arthritis this thin inner skin swells and becomes inflamed. The inflammation in turn may cause the capsule of the joint to become distended. The capsule, which surrounds the joint, consists pri-

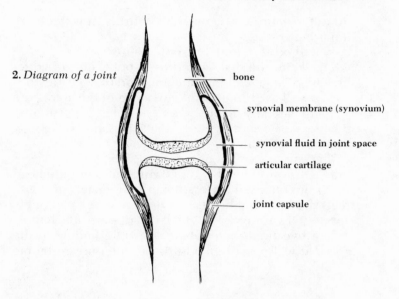

2. *Diagram of a joint*

bone

synovial membrane (synovium)

synovial fluid in joint space

articular cartilage

joint capsule

marily of connective tissue. *The pain in arthritis is mostly due to the stretching and twisting of the ligaments and capsules.*

THE SPINAL COLUMN

□ Between every two vertebrae of the spinal column (fig. 3) we find a thin disk with a gelatinous core. These disks permit the spinal column to be flexible, to rotate and to bend in various directions, much like the other joints of the body.

The joints of the body, as well as the vertebrae of the spinal column, which act like joints, are stabilized by ligaments and muscles. One part of the joint range is stabilized mostly by muscle action, the other part by ligaments, which act to prevent the joint from dislocating. The ligaments become stretched, weak, and pain-

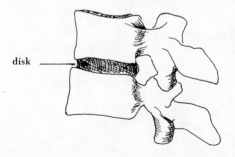

disk

3. *A resilient disk between each two vertebrae absorbs shock and permits the spine to flex.*

ful in the course of rheumatoid arthritis. It is therefore important to keep the muscles in good tone so that they will be able to stabilize the joints.

Thanks to the disks interposed between the vertebrae, the spinal column can be flexed (fig. 4). Flexibility, as well as stiffness and curvature of the spine, are again dictated by ligaments and muscles. The stronger the ligaments and muscles that cross the vertebrae, the more resilient the spine can be.

The cervical spine, or neck, consists of seven vertebrae. It is quite flexible, to permit motion of the head in all directions. The less flexible thoracic spine protects the lung and heart. It consists of twelve strongly supported vertebrae, to which the ribs are attached.

The five lumbar vertebrae form the hollow of the spine at waist level. In adulthood, the nine vertebrae

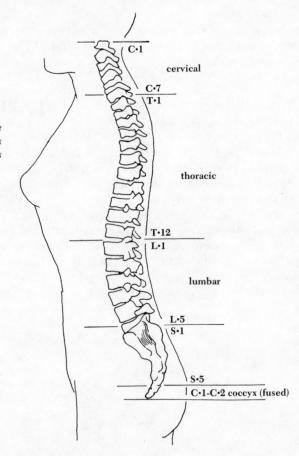

4. Side view of the spine and its various regions

C·1

cervical

C·7
T·1

thoracic

T·12
L·1

lumbar

L·5
S·1

S·5
C·1-C·2 coccyx (fused)

at the lower end of the spine fuse to form two inflexi-
ble structures. These are the sacrum, at the back of the
pelvis, and the coccyx, the tail end of the spine.

The curvature and the flexibility of the spine, together with the action of the powerful muscles that
overlie the back, combine to provide a certain degree
of springiness on impact. This gives protection to the
spinal cord, which passes through the hollow spaces
of the vertebrae, and to the brain, which sits in the
cranium at the top of the spinal column. For this springiness to remain effective, however, the muscles of
the back must be equal to the task of holding the
vertebrae in place. I have experienced utter discomfort riding in a car or a train soon after several weeks
of bed rest, during which time all muscles had been
reduced in strength. When bumpiness is not equili-
brated by the back muscles there is movement of the
vertebrae, which produces irritation of the nerves emanating from the spinal column.

The cervical spine and the lumbar spine are more
flexible than the thoracic spine between them, to
which the rib cage is attached. The section below the
lumbar spine, the sacrum, is stiff. The vertebrae adjacent to the stiffer parts of the spine, particularly the
seventh cervical vertebra and the fifth lumbar vertebra
seem to be especially sensitive; they are often the
sites of pain in arthritis.

Sudden, overly strong compression of vertebrae in
the flexible lumbar spine, or slight dislocation produced by the irregular pull of back muscles, can trigger a nasty irritation of nerves. This condition, known
as *sciatica*, must be carefully treated by rest to relax
the muscles, and then by exercises to strengthen the
muscles and retain flexibility. This is not a typical
symptom of rheumatoid arthritis, but I have experienced it in connection with involvement of one hip,
which caused asymmetrical stresses on the lower
spine.

THE MECHANICS OF SHOCK ABSORPTION

☐ When we walk, run, or jump, shock absorption is
supplied first through the resilience of two arches of
the foot—the metatarsal arch and the longitudinal
arch. Additional resiliency is supplied through the
muscles controlling the ankle joint.

The flexion and extension of the knee, controlled by the degree of tautness of the quadriceps muscle (extensor, fig. 5) also has a spring-like effect. The structures in the hip joint, particularly the cartilage, absorb the remaining impact, which is then transmitted to the fifth lumbar vertebra, just above the pelvis.

It is evident that shocks absorbed by a hip joint will result in some slight using-up of cartilage. In a healthy, young body, the cartilage is replaced, but as we grow older, our ability for this type of self-repair diminishes. If the stress on this joint is considerable, it may eventually result in reduced joint space and, finally the need for hip replacement surgery.

It is understandable, from the biomechanical analysis above, why sports that place severe stress on the hip and knee, such as jogging, constitute a risk when engaged in at an age when osteoarthritis is likely to occur, starting with the fourth decade of life.

Keeping the lumbar spine and the cervical spine straight places the least amount of stress on nerves emanating from these sections of the spinal cord. These are very important, large nerves. The sciatic nerve travels from the lumbar spine down to the legs and feet; other nerves travel from the cervical spine to the arms and hands. Irritation of nerve roots near the spine is likely to produce pain, not only in the back, but all through the extremities.

After one has been standing for a long time, the muscles of the back and neck become fatigued and they cannot act powerfully enough to stabilize the vertebrae and protect the nerve roots from irritation. We should therefore hold the lumbar spine, as well as the

5. *Skeletal muscle function*

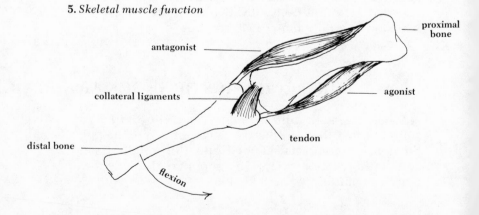

cervical spine, as straight as possible. This posture will help prevent lower back pain and discomfort arising from the neck.

VULNERABLE JOINTS IN ARTHRITIS

□ Figure 1 indicates the joints that are usually involved in arthritis. In order to avoid confusion, I do not mention all individual joints but concentrate on those most important for the purposes of exercise.

A few joints are predisposed to osteoarthritis, such as the distal interphalangeal joints of the fingers. The joints that are mostly involved in rheumatoid arthritis are the proximal interphalangeal joints and the metacarpophalangeal joints (big knuckles). In the acute phase of the disease inflammation can be expected in several of the big knuckles. The corresponding joints in the feet, the metatarsophalangeal joints, are often similarly involved.

(In my case of rheumatoid arthritis practically every single joint in the body has been involved at some time or another, except for the spine. For a time, cervical spondylitis [inflammation around the vertebrae] was suspected due to my long-drawn-out difficulties with the neck. However, as I describe it in chapter six, the difficulty was mainly due to tightened muscles, and eventually it subsided completely.)

As we grow older, calcium deposits grow around our vertebrae. The disks also become thinner. The resulting lowered flexibility, together with tight muscles, can produce strong pain. I consider these conditions only indirectly connected with rheumatoid arthritis, but the measures used to combat them can also be applied to arthritis: relaxation through heat, and exercise to free the muscles from metabolic waste products that produce pain.

Frequently in rheumatoid arthritis the symmetrical joints—the same joints on either side of the body—are involved simultaneously. In osteoarthritis the involvement is more often one-sided, possibly due to increased stress on a single joint.

In the later stages of rheumatoid arthritis, osteoarthritis is superimposed. Although it is not clear whether the process in my hip is rheumatoid arthritis or osteoarthritis, the same types of exercises and physical treatment are indicated. Shortening of the range of motion and weakening of the muscles around the joint are common complaints in both types of arthritis.

WHICH TYPE OF ARTHRITIS?

☐ My hip problem demonstrates the shortcomings of X-rays in diagnosing rheumatoid versus osteoarthritis. In the case of osteoarthritis, X-rays may not reflect the severity of the disability.

X-rays form only one part of the diagnostic criteria (established by a conference of international rheumatism associations) used in rheumatoid arthritis. Other criteria include swelling and redness of joints; sedimentation rate and other blood tests, such as hemoglobin; fatigue; morning stiffness; reduction of range of motion of various joints; reduced strength of hand grip; and functional complaints. A certain percentage of the criteria has to be positive in order to confirm the diagnosis of rheumatoid arthritis.

THE MUSCLES

☐ The muscles that move the bones are called *skeletal muscles*. They originate on a proximal bone and are usually inserted into a distal bone, which is moved by the muscle tendon. Figure 5 shows how muscles connected to a set of bones are pulling the distal bone into flexion.

The muscle pulling in the desired direction is called the *agonist*. The muscle pulling in the opposite direction is called the *antagonist*. Some muscles are called *synergists;* they aid in completing the desired motion. The antagonist muscles have the important function of stabilizing the joint so that the agonist does not pull it apart. They also hinder the too rapid and forceful contraction of the agonist, especially as the joint approaches the limit of its range. This hindering action is a learned reflex, information for which is stored in the spinal column. Observe how the toddler walks. He would like to walk in a straight line like the grownup, but he does not quite succeed at first. He learns to walk in a straight line. The coordination necessary for this is based on learned reflexes which keep him from overshooting his gait to one side or the other. Walking in a straight line, then, is coordinated through a reflex. That is why sleepwalkers walk straight in their sleep.

A NATURAL DEFENSE AGAINST PAIN

☐ When we suffer pain, we develop (or learn) new reflexes, namely those for defending ourselves against the pain. The pain in arthritis usually arises as we move our joints to the end of their range, and so we try to stop the motion before we reach that point. We do this by setting up new reflexes in the antagonist muscles.

If you have ever had bursitis in your shoulder, you'll recall that you were unable to raise your arm all the way. Your physician advised you to move the arm as much as possible once the pain decreased, so that the arm would not be limited in its motion after the episode of bursitis. If you tried to raise your arm during the painful period, the antagonists came forcefully into play to prevent your arm from reaching the painful range.

If you hold your arm long enough in the "defensive" position, short of reaching the painful range, a new reflex is learned. In a way, such defensive reflexes are welcome. They permit us to sleep at night, for example, by keeping us out of painful positions. Sometimes the antagonist muscles are so forcefully contracted that they go into defensive spasms just to protect us from the pain. In arthritis the pain is liable to last much longer than in bursitis.

During an acute attack of bursitis, which usually lasts only a few days, we are usually told to do some pendulum exercises (fig. 6). We swing the arm like a pendulum, without any muscle contraction. As long as the antagonist and the agonist muscles are not contracted, the antagonist muscle does not get any signals from the tiny neuromuscular bodies to stop the movement. These neuromuscular bodies, called *muscle spindles*, transmit their signals when they are compressed within a tense muscle. If the muscle is not contracted, as in a pendulum motion or in a passive movement of the arm by a therapist, the antagonist can be "cheated" and the arm can move beyond the point at which it would normally stop, due to the newly learned defensive reflex.

Passive exercise has its limitations. It is not practical

6. *Pendulum exercise: Swing arm lightly forward and backward or sideways or swing it in a circle.*

for everyday use, since it requires the cooperation of a therapist or assistant. The pendulum exercises which work well for the arms and legs, cannot be adapted for every joint in the body.

THE VALUE OF WARM-UP

□ The second, preferred way to "cheat" the muscle spindles is by relaxing the muscles through a warm-up. We know that athletes need warm-up exercises before they perform in an athletic event. This relaxes the muscles and makes them less liable to strain or sprain once strenuous and violent motion begins. The raised temperature within the muscle dampens the sensitivity of the muscle spindles, which are responsible for tenseness and tightness toward the end of the range of movement. The warm-up is usually accomplished by many repeated motions without overexertion.

The term *warm-up* is well chosen, since it actually means warming the muscles internally. A seldom mentioned fact is that the heat to maintain our body temperature above the ambient temperature is mostly generated within our muscles. A large quantity of blood flows through our muscles, carrying oxygen attached to hemoglobin. The oxygen is used for a chemical process within the muscle to produce contraction. Some of the energy is transmitted as mechanical energy through the tendons to move the distal joints (fig. 7); some also is used up in the muscle and produces heat. Think of the automobile, which uses up the gasoline mixed with air (oxygen) in the carburetor, and burns the mixture in the motor, producing mechanical motion to drive the car and also waste heat which is cooled off by air or water. If the car idles, no energy is transformed mechanically and the waste heat accu-

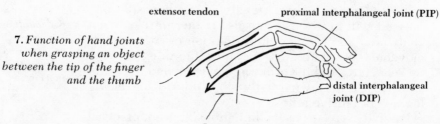

7. Function of hand joints when grasping an object between the tip of the finger and the thumb

extensor tendon

proximal interphalangeal joint (PIP)

distal interphalangeal joint (DIP)

flexor tendon

mulates more quickly. You have probably seen how a car overheats in stalled traffic in summertime. This process is in some way similar to the isometric contraction of the muscle, since here no energy is transformed into motion. All energy is converted to heat within the muscle.

The fact that warm-up really helps to relax the muscles has been shown by clinical observations. It can easily be seen that when starting out with fairly stiff muscles, as on awakening in the morning, we can extend the range of the shoulders by raising arms many times, say, ten to fifteen times. You will also easily notice that a warm bath is relaxing. It may increase your body temperature one to two degrees Fahrenheit (one-half to one degree Celsius), and you will need fewer repetitions of arm-swinging to get to the fullest possible range. Athletes who train in Florida and other warm places regain their fitness sooner because they need less warm-up.

I have found a PNF (proprioceptive neuromuscular facilitation) exercise technique very efficient to help stretch a joint to the limit of its range of motion. A technique, called "hold-relax," is used by therapists in this way: They exercise the antagonist muscle for several seconds (isometrically against resistance offered by the therapist), let the muscle relax, then move the limb to extend the limit of range.

Understanding the physiological basis of warm-up helped me to modify the well-proven PNF technique to home use. Once I was able to interpret the hold-relax technique as a *warm-up-and-relax* technique, I found I could substitute an isometric exercise in form of *muscle-tensing*, for straining against the resistance offered by a therapist. It should be noted that this type of *muscle-tensing* without accompanying motion, is coming into wider use as a general relaxation technique. Many of the exercises in this book employ this concept.

CIRCULATION AND THE ROLE OF THE LYMPHATIC SYSTEM

☐ In order for the muscles to become warm and to function well, we need increased *circulation*. Circulation means blood being pumped by the heart out through the arteries and into the muscles; the blood carries the necessary oxygen to generate heat, as well as nourishment for the process of cell replacement inside the muscles. Circulation also means blood being pumped out of the muscles through the veins, blood whose oxygen has been used in the process of burning the organically bound carbon; the residue is united with hemoglobin and carried away in the form of carbon dioxide. In the lungs, the carbon dioxide is eliminated from the blood (as in the exhaust of a car) and replaced by oxygen (as in the carburetor) from the air we breathe.

Circulation also means pumping out of the muscle metabolic waste products other than carbon dioxide —for instance lactic acid, which is removed through the lymphatic system and the veins. When lactic acid is left to accumulate in muscles, they become painful and stiff and tend to retain water. Let us find out why this accumulation of metabolic waste takes place, and how we can promote the healthy process of waste removal so as to avoid pain and stiffness. The muscles, as you will see, play a reciprocating role in this process.

The insides of the veins are equipped with little flaps, which allow the blood to move in one direction only. The flow is kept up partly due to the pumping action of the heart, as well as by compression of the veins by the muscles (one speaks of the "muscle pump").

The lymphatic system at first appears to be less ingeniously designed. Whereas the capillary endings of the arteries are intermittently intertwined with the corresponding venous capillaries, producing relatively little resistance to the flow of blood between the two systems, the lymphatic vessels collect their liquid and waste rather loosely from all the nooks and crannies of the body and get no push from the arterial system.

The lymphatic system, among its other duties, picks up particles which enter the body through the skin and which have to be prevented from entering the bloodstream lest they cause mechanical obstruction or infection in some of the organs. When someone is bitten by an insect, for example, the lymphatic system sets up a defense. Bacteria and viruses can be deposited in the skin through the insect bite together with solid particles of the insect's stinger. These are picked up by the lymphatic system in a dense network of flexible tubes equipped with flaps similar to those of the veins. The tubes cannot serve every single tiny spot of the skin. Therefore, a small pressure differential (suction) from the distal end of the tubes collects the wastes, including particles and bacteria. If the lymphatic system is unable to collect the bacteria, the bacteria will produce a localized infection with inflammation; a pimple forms which eventually bursts, thus eliminating some wastes directly from the body.

A similar process happens with solid particles which are too large to be absorbed by the lymphatic system. Think of a wooden splinter. If you permit the skin to heal over the splinter, white blood cells will start to fight against the intruder, as evidenced by pus and swelling. When the splinter is removed, the lymph continues to remove any debris and swelling. Waste travels through the tubes to the next lymph node in the network. These nodes are little organs located in places such as the elbow, neck, knee, and groin. Lymphocytes, white blood cells which abound in lymph nodes, fight intruding bacteria which are digested in order to bring them into a shape which will be harmless when they enter the bloodstream. The various lymph tubes collect into larger pipes as they move proximally, and these eventually empty into a large vein. Some poisons, rattlesnake venom, for instance, may not be stopped at a lymph node. If circulation is not stopped by a tourniquet and the poison sucked out at the point of entry, it may spread throughout the bloodstream and cause severe illness. Some viruses, like that of sleeping sickness, can completely immobilize a lymph node so that no liquid can pass through it, resulting in a swollen arm or leg.

The importance of maintaining good lymphatic circulation is obvious. To keep the lymph flowing, the system relies on the compressing action of the muscles and on the little flap valves within the lymph tubes. In the extremities, circulation of lymph is accomplished by the motion of the arms and legs. In the torso, it is helped along by breathing, namely by the muscle action of the diaphragm, the intercostal muscles, and the various other muscles that expand and contract the rib cage. Some lymph tubes ride piggyback on arteries and benefit from the pulsation of the blood through the arteries. The lymph flow is also increased by stronger blood flow, which can be encouraged by applying heat to the skin or rubbing it with a counterirritant ointment such as Ben-Gay, which helps to increase circulation.

If skin temperature is lowered slightly, lymph flow will be decreased near the skin. When a stye forms, which is an infection at the root of an eyelash caused usually by some dust or other particle, you are usually told to apply warm compresses. I have been able to make a stye vanish by applying compresses at the outset. This is due to the speed-up of the lymph drainage. Once the stye is in full bloom, however, the warm compress will help to open the stye and let the infection drain. This demonstrates the importance of maintaining warm skin temperature to keep the lymph flowing. (Some amphibious animals, like frogs, which spend time submerged in cold water, have special lymph hearts to help them maintain their lymph circulation.)

Fluid from the joints, specifically the joints of hands and feet, also drains through the lymphatic system, passing through delicate passages to the lymph vessels of the skin. It seems to follow from this that elimination of fluid from the joints will be enhanced by increasing circulation in the skin. Here we arrive at the relevance of this discussion for arthritics. It is very important that we become aware of how our lymphatic system functions in order to understand better the various physical therapy modalities available for treating our arthritic discomforts.

It is known that in rheumatoid arthritis the circulation becomes sluggish. This may have to do, in part at least, with the fact that arthritics make less use of their muscles; they move about less to avoid joint pain. Since most body heat is produced within the muscles, the temperature balance in the arthritic shifts somewhat in the direction of decreased surface temperature. (Cold hands and feet are often reported by arthritics. I myself have noticed a feeling of cold around my ankles, knees, and hips. For a while I felt this also on the shoulders, but the discomfort in these joints disappeared after a series of mud-pack treatments. I protect my ankles by wearing woollen socks of suitable weight in both summer and winter. I wear woollen knee warmers and woollen underwear or binders to protect flanks and hips. I find that I suffer considerably less pain in these various joints when I cover them with wool.)

Just as it disposes of viruses, bacteria, and particles from the skin, the lymphatic system also removes such items from the joint spaces. Viruses and bacteria may enter the joint space through the bloodstream, and the lymph system has to remove them in order to prevent a localized infection and inflammation. The job of the lymph system can be compared to that of a filter in which the undesirable particles are withdrawn from circulation and kept immobilized. Solid particles of ground-up cartilage are likely to appear in a joint space; in some cases, the particles may even be bone ground up through the movement of the joint. Once the lymph spaces and channels around a joint are damaged through inflammation, lymph clearance becomes more difficult. At such times, heat and muscle action are helpful to increase the flow of lymph from around the joints, thereby decreasing pressure and pain. I noticed that very strong heat often has an immediate (but not necessarily permanent) effect in removing pain, particularly in the feet, hands, and hips. The gentle warmth of a heating pad had very little effect. With hands and feet, I have obtained best results by using a whirlpool bath. For the hip, a Hydrocolator pack or, at home, application of a towel dipped into very hot water works best. Gentle heat, on the other hand, is indicated for the lower back, as very strong heat there might irritate nerves which emanate near the vertebrae. I find hot mud packs, a treatment available at certain spas, to be the best treatment for shoulders and knees. The effect of heat can be prolonged by the application of Ben-Gay or similar liniment.

Atmospheric pressure also has an influence on the functioning of the lymphatic system. Arthritics generally do not feel well when the barometric pressure decreases, as before a storm. It is noteworthy that increasing the pressure uniformly on the skin, with stretch gloves or an ace bandage, for example, makes arthritics feel more comfortable.

FOR BETTER LYMPHATIC ACTION

☐ A perfect modality to increase lymphatic drainage is the combination of heat and massage in the form of a very warm whirlpool bath. Just as normal people get improved well-being from these baths, arthritics can expect the special benefit of relief from pain. To take full advantage of the massaging action, you may want to maneuver yourself directly into the stream of the jets, but be careful, because the force may be too powerful for comfort. I have found that the small whirlpool for hands and feet, or the unit which is fastened to the tub, can be controlled well for my individual needs, regarding temperature as well as strength and direction of the jet.

Lymphatic drainage is important in arthritis not only for the joints but also for the muscles. If the skin above the muscle cools suddenly, we get a chill in the area, which might produce a muscle spasm, such as lumbago in the lower back. But any muscle may be painful when lymphatic drainage does not remove the metabolic waste products of muscle activity. The so-called charley horse is a case of a muscle being overstrained so that the lymph cannot remove the waste quickly enough. In the arthritic, lymph drainage will be sluggish and produce pain or stiffness even with minimal or no use of the muscles. The typical morning stiffness may be at least partially due to the fact that the lymph system is sluggish and requires some additional impetus to increase circulation, like a warm bath and some moving about.

You are aware that when you get up in the morning your feet are usually slightly swollen. Your shoes feel a little tight at first when you put them on. If you use bedroom slippers for a while, the feet will unswell due to the pumping action of the muscles within the legs, which circulates the fluids upward. Don't be surprised if this effect is particularly pronounced in arthritis.

I have gone into some detail regarding possible interconnection between lymphatic function and the symptoms of an arthritic, and the significance these interconnections may have for certain types of physical treatments. I have never come across this subject in any other book on the subject of arthritis. The reason for this lack, I suspect, is that the lymphatic system is very difficult to monitor. Only recently, with the advent of radioisotope tracing techniques, has it been possible to determine the speed of lymph flow. Slow clearance of lymph from joints of patients with rheumatoid arthritis, as compared with patients with osteoarthritis, has been observed by modern X-ray techniques. I have reported some facts about the working of the lymphatic system as described in physiology textbooks, and I have made my own inferences in order to have a working hypothesis to serve as a basis for various physical therapy modalities.

Of ten physicians whom I have approached with this hypothesis, I have found only two who were interested in studying it further. One is a radiologist and the other a specialist in nuclear medicine. Physicians with this type of expertise have available to them the necessary measurement systems for checking this hypothesis. Rheumatologists and physiatrists are reluctant to engage in such speculation before they see evidence. I mention this hypothesis, however, because it seems to me to account for a range of clinical symptoms and has helped me to develop a rationale to explain the effectiveness of certain treatment such as heat and massage. (As I said above, evidence of slow lymphatic clearance from rheumatoid arthritic joints already is available. See Resnick, D., in the Bibliography.)

I hope that I have helped to increase the understanding of some aspects of physiology, so that you can plan how to deal better with your arthritis.

3 Understanding Exercise

□ Body exercises are meant to increase or maintain our strength, flexibility, and endurance. All body movements are helpful in this regard, at least to the extent that without such movements we become weaker and stiffer, and we lose endurance. This happens especially after extended bed rest.

Many people exercise for a particular purpose. Out of the unlimited number of possible body motions they select those that are most efficient in producing the desired flexibility and development. The piano player practices for several hours each day to adapt his fingers and arms to the task of playing for several hours in a concert without becoming tired, which would interfere with his coordination and result in a poor performance; his fingers are nimble and strong. Body builders lift barbells of ever increasing weight and hold them up for ever longer periods of time as a way of developing muscle bulk. When they "present" themselves, you see arm, chest, and shoulder muscles of remarkable size. However, due to their bulk, body builder's muscles are not very flexible. Ballet dancers achieve great flexibility by means of deliberate exercise. Their muscle bulk is strongest in their lower extremities because of the demands that dancing places on their legs. Yoga practitioners exercise to stretch all parts of the body to the possible limit, achieving a high degree of flexibility and relaxation. Joggers develop strong leg muscles and endurance (cardiac reserve).

For the arthritic, many of the above mentioned examples are not appropriate since they would place too much stress on the joints (as in jogging or weight-lifting). But the same physiological principles of adaptation can be applied. An array of successful exercise techniques, tested and refined at various rehabilitation centers, allows the arthritic a choice of exercises.

In order to communicate well with your therapist or physician regarding such exercises, it is good to learn some of their names and some of the concepts involved.

A typical *active isotonic exercise* against resistance is a strengthening exercise for quadriceps using ankle weights. In such an exercise, you sit on a table and lift the legs individually as many times as possible with a particular weight. If you can exceed ten or twenty times, you switch to a heavier weight. This is also called a *progressive resistance exercise.* An *active isometric exercise* for the quadriceps might also use ankle weights, but the many repetitions are avoided. Instead, after one or two movements through the full range, the weighted ankle is held out with the knee extended as long as possible. Both methods, active isotonic as well as isometric, produce good results in muscle strengthening, although the isometric method has the advantage of being more gentle to the joints and less time-consuming. Later in this chapter I will give the physiological explanation for these methods in greater detail.

For rheumatoid arthritis, the usual recommendation regarding exercise is to start with isometric exercises as early as possible during a flare-up. However, active exercise, requiring motion of the joint against resistance and even against gravity (example: raising arms or legs), usually is encouraged only in quieter phases of rheumatoid arthritis. I have found that active-resistance exercises have been a strain on my joints throughout the course of the disease, and I am trying to substitute isometrics for pure strengthening.

Many of the exercises in part 2 produce strengthening with a minimum of strain on the joints. Note that many of them are done while you are lying on a bed. The bed, to some degree, reproduces the effect of buoyancy, thus reducing fatigue. These exercises are particularly helpful to those who are trying to build up strength after a period of bed rest. As stamina and muscle strength return, more time can be spent exercising in a sitting or standing position.

Active isotonic exercises with the lightest possible load and the largest number of repetitions, are, I find, the most advantageous for weak muscles. They also increase local circulation and exercise muscle fibers in that part of the range in which isometrics are not fully effective.

When I cannot do muscle tensing (setting) on a specific set of muscles, I find it beneficial to move the limbs repeatedly, even if just a little bit. Often, muscle tensing (setting) can then follow.

STRETCHING

□ Stretching muscles—for instance, stretching arms and legs and yawning—is something we often do on awakening, the way a cat stretches when it awakens from a nap. This is healthy, instinctive behavior, and something we should do regularly. Physiologically, stretching is good for arthritics: first, because it keeps the muscles at optimum length for highest efficiency (the cat needs to stretch before a long jump); second, because it keeps the joints loose by preventing muscle tightness; and third, because it helps reduce the chance of developing deformities as a result of abnormal muscle pull in combination with joint destruction.

Exercises to move the limbs as far as possible are called "range-of-motion exercises" (ROM) by physical therapists. When therapists speak of "stretching," they mean the same movements carried out passively beyond the range normally achieved by active motion without the therapist's help. In this stretching, the therapist moves the limb or other part of the body through its former range and slightly beyond without help from the patient.

It is usually not recommended that the patient carry out such passive exercises himself, since he may not be able to judge when he is exceeding the tolerable limit of pain, something therapists are trained to observe. I have adopted some therapists' techniques and have translated them into active exercise for the patient. I prefer to call them "stretching" even though no passive stretching is involved.

RANGE OF MOTION

☐ You should be very clear about the meaning of the words *full range of motion*. The purpose of daily exercises is to maintain our original, normal range of motion. With the arm, for instance, we move the arm straight over the head, out to the side, down, and backward as far as possible. These daily exercises are a preventive measure. Once the range has been noticeably reduced, which we see by our reduced function and may have confirmed by a therapist, we have to do *therapeutic* exercises for that particular part of the body. The task becomes more difficult and time-consuming, but it pays off by helping to prevent deformity, maintain function, and lessen pain. The slightest decrease in range is the signal for you to start corrective exercises.

DURING THE ACUTE STAGE

☐ In the *acute* phase of rheumatoid arthritis, when many joints are hot, swollen, and painful, it is particularly important to move all joints of the body at least once a day through the complete range of motion in order to prevent changes around the joint which are liable to occur at this time. The changes I refer to are *adhesions*, which, if not counteracted, may restrict the range of motion and lead to deformity that will interfere with function. Try to get help from a therapist at that stage to do passive exercises with you. Had I sought such help while in the acute stage, I think I would have avoided some of my present limitations. Arthritics are all too familiar with such limitations. The knee may not straighten out completely, which interferes with walking. You may be unable to make a complete fist, and so find it difficult to use a knife and fork properly. A restricted shoulder range, with a slightly bent elbow, prevents you from reaching for objects on a high shelf. If your neck is restricted in motion, you may not be able to turn your head to observe traffic when you are driving. Reduced ranges in the hip will slow down your walking and make it hard to climb stairs.

It takes much more effort and time to correct an adhesion or loosen a tightened muscle than to prevent these conditions in the first place. However, it is not easy to carry out stretching exercises in the acute stage, because of the pain. At this stage, pain is usually treated with medication and heat applications such as hot baths or compresses. The exercises should be done when pain is reduced, because then we achieve the greatest possible range.

BEGINNING PHYSICAL THERAPY

□ When treated properly with bed rest and medication, the acute period of rheumatoid arthritis should last no longer than one to two weeks. If you are in a hospital at that time, the therapists or nurses will carry out the necessary exercises with you, and toward the end of your hospital stay they will train you to do these exercises at home. Some patients become discouraged by what seems to them a very ambitious and exhausting regimen of exercise prescribed at that time. So many repetitions and such expenditure of effort! I felt that if I were to carry out these prescriptions, I would be able to do nothing else in my life but sleep, eat, and exercise. There would be no reserve energy left for work or for leisure activities.

I believe in a different approach to exercise, one in which you understand the exact rationale for each exercise so that you can tailor it to your own body needs. This approach uses the most modern techniques to increase the efficiency of the exercises and make them faster and less fatiguing to perform, with fewer repetitions. You will find it easier to motivate yourself to exercise daily and will have more time for your work and leisure activities. It is my aim in this book to provide such an approach.

ISOMETRICS AND ISOTONICS

□ We distinguish between *isometric* exercises, during which the joints are not moved, and *isotonic* exercises, during which joints are moved. During an *active* exercise, muscles are exerted. In a *passive* exercise, muscles are relaxed and parts of the body are moved, for instance, with the help of a therapist or by the force of gravity. Nerve signals from and to the muscles can be stimulated and controlled in such a way as to permit the widest possible range of motion of the joints. Yoga exercises are designed to achieve this, but the technique used in Yoga is not ideally suited to the conditions of arthritis, though it is very useful as a prophylactic measure when arthritis is not present. I have selected the proprioceptive neuromuscular facilitation technique, PNF, for this purpose.

PNF refers to the exercise techniques and patterns developed about thirty years ago for use with infantile paralysis patients. Some of these techniques have been modified to include isometric contractions to facilitate gains in range of motion, and are widely used by physical therapists with arthritic patients. I have adapted some of these techniques for home by using isometric muscle tensing (setting) rather than straining against an external resistance. As you become more aware of your own body and the individual muscle groups, you can learn to master the technique of isometric muscle tensing (setting). In this way you will not require the aid of a therapist or helper to furnish resistance for the isometric exercise to relax muscles prior to stretching.

Most of our body activities require a combination of isometric and isotonic contractions. For instance, handling objects consists mostly of adjusting the grasp of the hand (isotonic), then holding the object (isometric). In describing exercises, I use the words *isometric* or *isotonic*, depending on which type of contractions produce the effect for which the exercise was designed. For example, I consider use of barbells an isometric exercise if the weights are held for as long a period as possible overhead. If they are raised and lowered rhythmically, this is an isotonic exercise.

ISOMETRICS UPDATED

☐ Isometric exercises were the subjects of great public interest in the 1960s. All you had to do was to press your arms sideways against the frame of a door, your hands against a desk top, your legs against a chair, and so forth, for the brief "maximum" isometric contraction. This fad occurred after isometric training was analyzed scientifically in Germany in the middle 1950s. Interest waned when athletes and trainers could not confirm that isometric exercises consisting of only a few seconds of muscle contraction could re-place the much more time-consuming and strenuous training methods of the past.

In the meantime, scientific analysis has continued, and permits these efficient exercises to be utilized in a rational way. This is especially important in the management of arthritis, since isometric exercises are carried out without movement of any joint, or with very little movement. A number of works published in the last decade (see Bibliography) have given us a better understanding of how isometric exercises work, and how they can be done both efficiently and conveniently to obtain optimum results. A full understanding permits us to design our own set-up for exercise without blindly following instructions. Even though I will describe these exercises in cookbook detail, with proper understanding you can translate these same exercises into efficient exercises for any muscle group.

I want to come back to the importance of moving *all* joints once a day through their complete range, during the acute phase, in order to prevent adhesions, muscle imbalance, and deformity. Had I known in the first week of my disease that it was important to straighten out my knee once during the day, I could have easily done so and thereby avoided permanent damage. Although physical therapy—which largely means daily exercise—is not a cure for arthritis, it certainly can prevent needless crippling. About 80 percent of rheumatoid arthritis patients will be able to continue their regular activities and jobs if they exercise and continue their medical treatment. At least, such is the estimate given by Healey, Wilske, and Hansen in their excellent book, *Beyond the Copper Bracelet: What You Should Know About Arthritis* (see Bibliography).

Pain is always a limiting factor in exercise. For example, someone in an acute phase involving the shoulder will achieve less range of motion when moving the arm himself than when a therapist or helper moves the arm while the patient's muscles are relaxed. The important thing is the range you gain, not the effort you exert, nor the pain you suffer. Try to avoid pain and get the largest obtainable range from each joint—that is my prescription for a "stretching" exercise. I have seen in arthritis manuals the statement that pain is permissible so long as it doesn't persist for more than an hour. But how can you recognize whether pain is going to persist for an hour or more at the time that you induce it? I prefer to exercise just to the limit of pain and no further.

THE FORMULA FOR STRENGTHENING

☐ It is helpful to understand fully the physiological basis for exercises. Although you need not master the following explanation of muscle strengthening, you may find it surprising and informative reading nonetheless.

The principle involved in muscle strengthening is to stimulate the growth of the muscle fibers through a muscle contraction stronger than the one used in normal activities. One daily *maximum contraction* of one second permits the muscle to gain its maximum possible strength within six weeks. One daily maximum contraction of six seconds shortens the time to about five weeks; several daily maximum contractions, for a total of thirty seconds, achieve maximum strengthening in four weeks, and one daily contraction at two-thirds of maximum strength lasting one second requires eight and one-half weeks to arrive at maximum strength. These results were reported for normal people starting with 80 percent of their strength potential. This means they added 20 percent strength and reached their limit in from four weeks to eight and a half weeks, depending on the frequency, length, and power of the daily contractions.

The question arises here: *What is a maximum contraction?* According to Müller, a maximum muscular effort is one that cannot be maintained for more than about twelve seconds. It corresponds to about three times the strength at which a muscle is normally used. Double the normal strength produces a fair degree of isometric strengthening, even though it is not quite as strengthening as maximum effort. A one-time daily effort of two to three seconds, at maximum strength, is supposed to produce the biggest possible result in strengthening. Exercising at twice the normal effort (equivalent to two-thirds of the maximum effort) requires six seconds of effort, which can be distributed over several periods, for instance, two times at three seconds (count of six) each.

In the paper, " 'Hand Gym' for Patients with Arthritic Hand Disabilities: Preliminary Report, 1978" (see Section 4 in Bibliography), a strength increase of about 20 percent was reported for the average of finger muscles after sixteen weeks. The exercises were done twice daily for two to three seconds (or a count of six by pressing fingers as strongly as possible against the sides or bars of the Hand Gym. These being unsupervised exercises, I estimate that patients probably exercised to one-half or one-third of their maximum strength. Isometric strengthening can be achieved, therefore, by exerting only twice the normal strength for two to three seconds daily. This is also the clinical recommendation of Dr. Theodor Hettinger, who, together with Dr. Müller, has laid the groundwork for our understanding of the rationale of isometric exercise, and it has shown itself to be quite efficient in finger exercises.

Theoretically, the same regimen of twice-daily exercises of two to three seconds' duration, contracting as strongly as possible (i.e., two to three times the normally used strength, being equivalent to one-third to one-half maximum strength), should be sufficient to exercise all other skeletal muscles. If the muscles are very weak due to prolonged nonuse, as after bed rest, their strength increase will be fairly rapid in the beginning and will slow down as you come closer to the potential limit.

When daily training is stopped, the gain will be lost again in about the same period of time that was required to reach it, unless exercises are continued at least once a week or once every two weeks. Even at this rate, the muscle strength will eventually settle at the limit dictated by the condition of our joints. The study with the Hand Gym showed that eighteen patients with rheumatoid arthritis gained about 20 percent in strength in four months and a satisfactory increase in function; the latter was due also to an increase in flexibility—that is, in the ranges of the small finger joints.

After four years, the eighteen patients with rheumatoid arthritis and five with osteoarthritis, who also went through the four months' training period, reported that they were satisfied with their strength and flexibility and hand function. Objective tests showed that the osteoarthritic patients had maintained half of the gain in strength after the four months' training period (double the flexibility range gain which they had achieved in the four months). The rheumatoid patients fell back to their original strength (maintained half their gain in range of flexibility). All the patients reported exercising with the Hand Gym during the four-year period—some once or twice a week, some once every two weeks, some daily when they felt they needed it. The average was once weekly.

I learned from this that exercises done once or twice weekly on a regular basis are of benefit to maintain strength. This conforms to the results of studies reported by Müller. He found that a one-time weekly isometric workout in normal persons helps to maintain strength required in the daily work, thereby preventing fatigue. Thus, if we give our muscles a workout on the weekend, it gets us well through the week. In addition, a yearly vacation of several weeks, during which our muscles get a good workout, tones us up for the year ahead.

Apparently, the longer the training period is, the longer the gain in muscle strength remains with us. It seems therefore unnecessary to exercise several times daily to a total of thirty seconds for each muscle. Two to three seconds (count of six) has been shown to be quite acceptable with finger muscles.

This, however, is not the case for some of the large muscles of the lower extremities and of the buttocks. These are very large and powerful muscles, as compared with the finger muscles. Also, they consist of several parts. The quadriceps, for instance, has four parts located at slight angles. In my experience, these complex and large muscles are best exercised with the full six-second maximum effort.

TECHNIQUES OF MUSCLE CONTRACTION

□ So far we have discussed the duration of the contractions and the force required for efficient isometric strengthening. We must also consider the various ways of exerting muscle power. The usual direction is to press against a strong resistance—an immovable object or the resisting hand of a helper or therapist. It is also possible to contract, or tense ("set"), the muscles without straining against any external resistance (as when the body builder flexes his arm to display a bulging biceps); this technique is highly useful in exercising the quadriceps.

The resisting hands of a therapist or helper are ideal. They are infinitely adjustable to the various directions in which the parts of the body have to be pressed to obtain the desired muscle contractions. Also, they permit a very slight motion of the joints so that signals are transmitted to the spinal cord and brain, which actuate stronger muscle contraction. But when no therapist or helper is available, it is still possible to exercise isometrically. A solid piece of furniture or a doorframe can present an "infinitely" strong resistance, though it will not be as conducive to generating a very strong muscle contraction as are the helper's hands.

Certain authors (e.g., Swezey; see Bibliography) recommend using a belt or a beach ball. I found both of these very useful. The beach ball is inflated to permit a slight amount of "give." When it is squeezed between the legs, for instance, you will notice a stronger contraction on the inside of the thighs than when you push your knee against a table leg. The belt can be a regular leather or plastic belt with buckle. An elastic belt is probably still better, but is more difficult to obtain. With the belt looped around your arms, spreading the arms apart permits a slight movement of the joints due to the elasticity of the arm muscles. (Details will be given where the exercises are described.)

I have found that after carrying out isometric exercises a number of times against resistance, it was possible for me to do muscle tensing (setting) exercises for most of the other muscles of the body. This may be easier for some people than for others. (It took me quite a while before I could tense my calf muscles without standing on my toes.) But it is important to acquire this ability, especially if a particular movement is painful for you. For example, it may be difficult for you to stand on your toes because of a painful metatarsal. Another reason to learn muscle tensing (setting) is that once you master the technique you can exercise at almost any time and place, quite apart from your regular morning and evening exercise periods, for instance when sitting on a chair watching TV.

Since I learned muscle tensing for the various muscles, I have used this method for increasing strength and building stamina, as well as for relaxation following the muscle contraction.

SLOW AND FAST TWITCHES

☐ Isometric exercises for warm-up and relaxation do not have to be exercises of maximal effort, of three or six seconds' duration. They can be, for instance, several contractions, one to two seconds long, during which blood is pumped into the muscle and all the work of the muscle is converted into heat within the muscle. Thus these "twitches" are highly efficient in obtaining relaxation due to heat with a minimum of effort.

I call the type of contraction just described, lasting from one to three seconds, a *slow muscle twitch*. (It is not to be confused with the neurological concept of muscle twitch generated through contraction of individual muscle fibers of very short [millisecond] duration.) The relaxation obtained may be used for stretching exercises to increase range of motion. The twitches put considerably less strain on the joints—indeed no strain at all—as compared with repeated motions of the extremities (arms and legs) to the limit of the range. These types of exercises can be useful at various parts of the range, in order to exercise some of the fibers that may have been omitted during the chief isometric exercise for the particular muscle.

In addition to the slow twitch, I have used to great advantage an exercise I call the *fast twitch*. This is fairly rapid, repetitive twitching. You can twitch as you count—1,2,3,4, etc. It should be forceful, but you should be able to repeat it at least twenty times before the muscle becomes fatigued. Gradually, this will build up endurance so that you can twitch with the same force twice as many times. This exercise helps improve local capillary capacity within the muscle, and thereby helps to build up endurance in function. Note, however, that deliberate exercises to increase cardiovascular activity are also needed for this endurance build-up.

The twitches are particularly useful as a first step in rebuilding strength. After a prolonged bed rest, I noticed my calf muscles, as well as the muscles of my left arm, were particularly weak and reduced in size. I tried to build them up with isometric exercises, but this was not very successful, since it required raising myself on the front part of the foot. I could not lift the heels off the ground even once. I thereupon started exercising the calf with a fast twitch. I did this several times a day, and, at the end of the first day, I could do twenty twitches before fatiguing. The second day, I could do fifty. I then tried lifting my heels and standing on the front part of the foot, and I could do it briefly five to ten times. I had a similar experience mobilizing the biceps of my left arm, which was at first so weak that it shuddered when I contracted it. Within two days of fast twitching exercises I could start lifting one- and two-pound weights.

Fast twitching the buttock muscles, as well as the thigh muscles, is a good warm-up for the effort of getting up from low chairs, beds, and the like. (By now, I have learned to avoid low chairs. I am always looking for the highest chair in any room I visit, and at home I use foam-rubber pillows to raise the seat height of chairs. This is after fifteen years of arthritis, when the hip and knee joints have deteriorated.)

I also use fast twitching to warm up feet and ankles when they get chilled and stiff during the winter.

SIMULATED JOGGING

□ After I practiced slow and fast twitching for some time, it occurred to me that many motions in sports, such as jogging and bicycle riding, involve slow and fast muscle-twitching, and that I could really practice "isometric jogging" and "isometric bicycling" by twitching various muscle groups in the proper sequence, just as if I were carrying out these sports. I found that it is best to do isometric bicycling when you sit down, and isometric jogging when standing. You cannot carry out a proper, forceful isometric contraction of your buttock muscles when sitting, so you don't get the same feedback from your body that you would in actual jogging. In bicycle riding, the force transmitted to the pedals starts with the knees bent, rather than nearly extended, as in jogging.

When I reported this "invention" of an exercise to my therapist, she told me that she does just this occasionally, and I know that she is an ardent jogger. Apparently when people do a sport, they like to play the same muscles when they relax. So if you have ever jogged or bicycled, or if you bicycle now, try the isometric sport sometime while watching TV. Please do not do actual jogging if you have arthritis! This may be too great a strain for your knee, hip, and ankle joints.

What to Do About Pain and Stiffness 4

☐ When we are young, we tend to dismiss pain, to suppress it mentally, or "tough it out." If it doesn't go away, we might take a couple of aspirins. After strenuous sports, we can usually heal our aches with a hot shower and a rubdown. We know that our bodies will repair themselves in time. If I suffered a sprained ankle when jumping or mountain climbing, I knew that a properly applied bandage would ease the pain and all would be well again in a few days.

When I contracted arthritis, however, I learned that pain could be excruciating, unlike anything I had known before—perhaps with the exception of a toothache. But an extremely painful joint cannot be treated like a tooth; it doesn't help to tough it out and take a couple of aspirin tablets.

It took me quite a few years after the onset of the disease to radically change my attitude toward pain. I started to understand that the self-repairing ability of the muscles, tendons, ligaments, and other structures around the joints is diminished in arthritis. I have learned to observe—even to anticipate—every little twinge of pain occurring near the joints, and to take the right physical measures to heal the hurt and to prevent it from becoming worse. In my youth I would have looked on such behavior as hypochondria. But now that I have rheumatoid arthritis I respect the first twinges of pain. I know that if the cause is not removed the twinges often develop into much more persistent pains.

I believe (based on my experience) that most arthritic pain develops slowly enough so that it can be nipped in the bud before it becomes excruciating and requires very powerful medications. The inability to deal preventively, or therapeutically, with pain after it has settled in produces disabilities and depression which may prevent us from taking effective measures to get back on our feet.

PROS AND CONS OF PAINKILLERS

☐ When the pain of arthritis is overwhelming, all one wants to do is reach for a painkiller. If you are using drugs in the management of pain, you will, of course, be doing so under the guidance of your physician. I do feel it can be helpful, though, to review certain of the other consequences—aside from freedom from pain —that go with the use of drugs. Often it comes as a surprise to arthritics that painkillers and other medications actually add to the stress in their lives and interfere with general healthy living.

The problem with painkillers is twofold. First, there are harmful side effects—slow stomach bleeding caused by aspirin ingestion, the narcotic effects of codeine, and the lasting and deleterious side effects of cortisone, which have now made it rare as a continuous treatment. Your physician will weigh these considerations carefully before prescribing medication, especially in the case of cortisone, which, when overused, can cause problems worse than the disease itself.

Furthermore, when an anti-inflammatory agent like cortisone is injected into a joint, it can produce a temporary pain-free euphoria during which we can seriously damage a joint. I once had a cortisone injection in my painful arthritic shoulder, after which I proceeded to saw a thick branch off a tree. The next day, the pain redoubled. It certainly *felt* as if I had damaged the joint.

Sleeping pills present yet a different problem, in that the effect of any one pill tends to be nullified after prolonged use, and this may lead to dependency. I agree that a good night's rest is essential for everyone, and especially for the arthritic, but I believe that purely physical means can go a long way toward inducing sound sleep. I discuss this at length in the next chapter. Try the tense-relax technique: tense each muscle consecutively for two seconds, relax, tense the next muscle, relax, and so on.

MUSCLE RELAXANTS

☐ Muscle relaxants are often prescribed for their relaxing and tranquilizing effects. One was prescribed for me by my rheumatologist in small doses, 2 mg. of Valium once or twice daily, and for some time I felt only beneficial effects. Once a month, on seeing my doctor, I was asked to report any untoward effects from the tranquilizers. It was during a vacation of several months, during which I didn't see a physician, that the accumulated side effect arrived, and it was very disagreeable: inability to concentrate, depression, changed personality. I stopped taking the tranquilizer, and after a few days these symptoms disappeared. The first day after stopping the tranquilizer was very difficult to live through. What I did that day, I can't recall. Evidently I have repressed the memory. All I know is that the day and night were a nightmare. The experience has reinforced my belief that it is better to use physical means to combat muscle tension. This means exercising regularly and arranging your life so that mental tension does not exceed your level of tolerance.

COMBATING CHRONIC PAIN

☐ In some cases of pain and disability, surgical intervention is required to reconstruct or replace misshapen or misaligned joints. Usually, pain disappears after such procedures, but sometimes it lingers on. Cases in which all rational treatment has been exhausted and pain still persists can be called chronic pain cases. Many chronic pain clinics have been established throughout the country to deal with these problems. Many of the modalities used in such clinics are available also from the rehabilitation departments of major hospitals. Some are very new and are not yet available everywhere. These include acupuncture and transcutaneous nerve stimulation (TNS). The latter is an electronic method of pain control which a patient can be taught to use at home. Other modalities include hypnosis and guided imagery, both of which are proving valuable in opposing pain through mind control.

In guided imagery the patient is taught to guide his imagination in pleasurable directions so that pain is displaced as a focus of attention. This brings to mind the case of Norman Cousins, former editor of the *Saturday Review,* who fought his case of otherwise intractable arthritis by setting up a deliberate program of viewing funny movies that would make him laugh for extended periods of time. The strategy succeeded, for reasons no one quite understands. I wonder if Mr. Cousins might have obtained some cleansing effect as the diaphragmatic and other muscular action associated with strong laughter stirred up his lymphatic system?

GETTING AT THE CAUSE OF PAIN

☐ I have used a great many of the available modalities in fighting my arthritis, including painkillers. During a bursitis attack that preceded the arthritis, I found that codeine allowed me to sleep. During my first strong flare-up of rheumatoid arthritis, I got relief from Butazolidin. At later stages I had cortisone injections into my finger joints and shoulder.

Learn, if you can, to anticipate painful episodes and to use physical means such as immobilization, heat, and exercise to deflect development of the pain. When I first read the principle that physical therapy ideally should be able to prevent a painful state, I did not understand it, nor did I believe it. Now, after fifteen years of arthritis, I have a fuller grasp of its meaning. I am trying to communicate in this book the various exercises and other modalities you can use to combat pain. I am grateful for all strong painkillers with which I was treated, and I acknowledge their value in decreasing pain and making it possible to increase range through exercise. But the less medication you use, and the more the pain is eliminated through physical means, the more comfortable you will be.

What I offer my readers is my optimism that something can be done to help alleviate and remove the cause of each hurt in any part of our body due to arthritis I have described, in the chapter on the neck and jaw, my experiences with serious disability and pain which dragged on for a year before it was cleared up. Had I been aware at the beginning of these involvements of their cause and the various modalities useful in their treatment, I am convinced that my period of suffering would have been radically reduced. Learning where the pain comes from helps us to decide how to deal with it. We will not always necessarily succeed with the first modality we try. But if one doesn't work, another one will.

TO REDUCE INFLAMMATION

□ Before discussing other modalities of pain management, let me repeat that most of the pain in rheumatoid arthritis is due to inflammation. The inflammation in the joint is accompanied by a considerable thickening of the synovium, the membrane that encloses the joint space. At the same time, there is a tendency for fluid to be retained in and around the joint. The pressure of the liquid and of the synovium against adjacent ligaments and against the capsule that surrounds the joint produces pain, as ligaments and/or the capsule are stretched and twisted. This produces pain. Inflammation also occurs along tendons that cross the joints. Tendons are covered by synovial sheaths, which are also liable to become inflamed, so that pain is felt at points along the tendon.

If the inflammation was not contained sufficiently by the drug regimen, as becomes evident from the pain, the following physical means are available to fight it: (1) rest, (2) heat, (3) gentle movements to dissipate stagnant liquid, and (4) exercises.

REST

□ Rest can be provided for joints or tendons in several ways. The painful joint or painful part of the tendon is immobilized by a splint or, if a splint is not available, by an Ace bandage. Immobilization is particularly useful overnight to prevent the slight movements during sleep that tend to irritate the joint. (Think of a broken bone. It will never heal if you simply rest in the hope of not moving it. You have to set it in a cast in order for it to heal.) The fact that immobilization helps has been amply described in medical literature. I have experienced its success and have described it in various parts of this book concerning hands, ankles, and knees. I have never read a satisfactory explanation for this effect. One factor contributing to inflammation may be the disturbance of the tiny lymph channels near the joints. Complete immobilization may help to restore efficient flow through these channels, and as liquid clears from the inflamed area, there is less pressure on pain-sensitive structures.

Morning stiffness is typical in arthritis. It is usually due to the accumulation of fluids in or near the joints during the night. The length of time it lasts after you arise is a good measure for the degree of activity of the disease. The reason it subsides after a while is that you move about after you get up, and the movements of the body tend to cause the accumulated fluids to dissipate. A warm bath in the morning during which you move about—using soap, rinsing and drying yourself—speeds up the disappearance of morning stiffness through the combination of heat and gentle motion. I feel the very important exercises to maintain and increase joint range should be done after the bath or after the morning stiffness has subsided in other ways, so that their main purpose—namely, moving your extremities through the largest range possible—will not be hindered.

Gelling, a lack of movement due to pain (a phenomenon similar to stiffness), can occur after you have been sitting without moving for a long time, especially in a draft. It can happen also if you have been clutching a telephone tightly during a lengthy conversation. You seem to have a hard time letting go of the receiver. If you notice gelling, make sure that you move frequently while you sit, especially your feet and ankles. Also, shift the telephone receiver from hand to hand several times during a long conversation. Gelling after long periods of sitting is not specifically indicative of arthritis. People generally are liable to become stiff if they sit for extended periods of time, for instance during air travel.

WHY REST AND EXERCISE?

☐ Here I will remind you of the chief reason why we exercise to obtain relief from pain. Through exercises we can keep a joint in proper alignment and so reduce the stress on ligaments. A joint is usually stabilized in part of its range by muscles and in another part by ligaments. If the joint is used in that part of the range which relies on muscle power, less stress is going to be placed on ligaments, therefore there will be less twisting or stretching of these ligaments (which are already weakened by the disease), and less pain.

The reader is justified in asking here, "Why are rest and movement both used to combat pain?" The answer is that they work in different ways. For reasons not yet fully understood, there seems to be some recovery from the process of deterioration during complete rest. When there is gentle movement, either active or passive, the flow of liquid through the larger lymph channels away from the joints is encouraged, thereby lessening pressure and promoting the removal of wastes. A muscle containing metabolic products like lactic acid, which have not been cleared away, feels very painful. In the athlete, such a condition can result after a peak performance like the one-hundred-yard dash. By slow, deliberate muscle action, these products are "pumped" out of the muscle, and that is why the athlete will run slowly in place for a time following an event. In the arthritic, such a condition arises when muscles go into spasm, working extra hard to protect a painful area. For instance, to prevent a vertebra from pinching a nerve, the muscle may contract to pull the vertebra to one side. In order for this muscle to be relieved of the metabolic product of this effort, it has to be exercised. But exercise may not be easy so long as the muscle is not relaxed. Relaxation can be achieved through heat (also through cold), massage, and immobilization of the concerned vertebra (for instance, by wearing a cervical collar).

Indirectly, pain can be produced when nerves are pinched or compressed due to the irregular pull of muscles and distortion of the supporting bones nearby. Such pain—for instance, sciatica pain in the lower back reaching down into the legs—can be very strong and disabling. Surrounding muscles have to be relaxed and exercised to reduce abnormal pulls.

All conditions of pain should be reported to your physician, so that you can decide together what modality to choose to combat it. Your physician also must make the extremely important determination of whether your pain is really caused by arthritis, or whether it comes from a pinched nerve or some completely different and unrelated condition. Sometimes these conditions are very difficult to tell apart.

WHAT HEAT CAN DO

☐ My rheumatologist told me at an early stage of my arthritis, "Heat is your best friend." An exact explanation of why heat works so well to reduce pain in arthritis has not yet been conclusively established. One theory suggests that the pain-nerve endings send fewer pain signals to the brain when they are either heated or cooled. This is why both heat and cold are usable modalities to reduce arthritic pain. However, both heat and cold, as they are administered for arthritis, also result in increased circulation, and this may have a salutary effect in clearing fluids from painful areas.

Most heat applications are either wet or dry. In the first type, water in some form—for example, a whirlpool bath or a steaming hot compress—is the conductor of the heat. Dry heat radiates from some nonhumid source, such as a heat lamp. Let us consider first the various applications of wet heat.

WATER THERAPIES

☐ *Thermal pools,* therapeutic pools the size of swimming pools with the water kept at approximately body temperature, are available in the United States at some rehabilitation centers and individual hospitals. (Swimming is generally not permitted in such pools to keep patients from bumping into one another.) There is always at least one therapist in attendance, who will assist you in a brief session of stretching exercises after the body is properly warmed up and the muscles relaxed. I found such treatment particularly useful for stretching the hamstring muscles. I could hold my leg upward, with the knee straight, at a right angle to the body. I found also hip abduction (spreading of legs) and hip extension considerably easier to carry out in warm water.

In one hospital I received hydrotherapy in a Hubbard tank, a large, round tub which permits exercising the legs and arms under water. This tank is equipped with several whirlpool attachments which permit the use of very warm water, so that greater muscle relaxation can be achieved.

Jacuzzis and pools of similar design can be found now at health clubs and even apartment buildings throughout the country. These feature strong jets of water or air which keep the pool well agitated, permitting the use of quite high water temperature—104° F (40° C)—without causing discomfort. The jet of water may be too strong to use directly on joints at close range for massage effect, but it is easy enough to sit or move out of the way of the jets and thereby get the beneficial effects these pools offer.

I liked the action of portable whirlpool attachments so much that I purchased one for use in my bathtub at home. The great benefit of installing a whirlpool is, again, the ability to use hotter bathing water (100° F), (38° C). The swirling water can be easily directed against feet, legs, and hips: it does not reach back and shoulders.

Note that when you come out of a warm bath at home, the room you enter next should be as warm as possible, definitely not below 72° F (22° C). (I use an auxiliary electric heater in my bedroom for this purpose.) Cool air after a hot bath is an invitation to muscle spasms and this completely defeats the benefit of the warm bath.

A hot shower is not likely to warm the body as much as a warm bath, but it does allow you to direct a hot stream of water against your shoulders and back. This provides a good massage as well as heat, especially if you have a shower head that can give a massaging action.

FOMENTATIONS

☐ Outside the bathroom I have used heat applications in the form of fomentations. For this you make a compress by dipping a folded towel in very hot water, then wringing it out and applying it over the joint. Cover it with a plastic sheet for insulation. Renew the compress about every five minutes. So that the skin does not cool off between applications, it is useful to work with two compresses, applying one immediately after the other one has cooled off.

ELECTRIC HOT PADS

□ A humid electric hot pad gives an effect somewhat similar to the hot compress. The pad I use, called the Thermophore, available in surgical supply stores (at about fifty dollars) is dry to start with, but sheds some humidity between the long, soft fibers of its cover while in use (the humidity, as I understand it, is extracted from the air). The pad gives out heat only while the pushbutton switch is kept depressed, and the heat is much stronger than with the usual type of electric heating pad.

Many automatic electric heating pads are equipped with a flat sponge which can be dipped into water for a wet application. They produce a moister but less warm application than the Thermophore. Electric hot pads do not conform as well as compresses to round joints such as the knee, shoulder, or elbow. They work better on flat areas, such as the back and hips. Remember that in case of trouble with the lower back, *mild* heat is usually recommended.

FOR PAINFUL HANDS

□ A treatment helpful for painful hands is soaking them for twenty minutes or so in hot water. I use a plastic bowl into which I run a slow but constant stream of water, as hot as I can stand it. I put about a half a cup of epsom salts into the bowl, which contributes to heat conduction and helps protect the skin.

To prolong the feeling of comfort after a heat application, it helps to apply a rubbing ointment or liniment containing salicylic acid, menthol, or camphor, ingredients which increase circulation.

The *paraffin* treatment for hands is usually administered in hospitals or clinics, since the heating of the paraffin has to be carefully supervised; it cannot be overheated or the patient may suffer burns. In this treatment, the hands are dipped completely into a hot paraffin bath. When the hands are withdrawn and cooled in the air, the thin layer of paraffin sets and hardens. The hands are dipped again briefly several times until a number of wax layers have built up, covering the hands like tight gloves. The hands with the paraffin "gloves" are then wrapped in a towel and rested for twenty minutes, after which the wax is removed. After such an application, my hands felt pleasantly warm and pain-free, but fairly stiff.

A soak in hot water leaves my hands flexible and I am able to move my fingers during the application. I find this preferable.

DRY HEAT

☐ Dry heat is another way of treating the pain of arthritis. In general I find heat lamps less efficient than wet applications. They produce localized hot areas on the skin which are susceptible to cool drafts, even in rooms at normal temperature. Dry heat from the sun, when taken in a dry climate, is extremely pleasant and makes the whole body feel good. In a humid climate sunbathing can be disagreeable, since the normal evaporation from the skin cannot take place due to the humidity. In addition, a draft or slight wind can produce cooling of localized perspired areas, and muscle spasms and further pain may result.

Diathermy and *ultrasound* also can be considered dry heat. They employ electromagnetic waves which are aimed inside the body. I had diathermy treatment prior to cortisone injections into the finger joints. The fifteen-minute treatment made my fingers feel warm and comfortable only while the application lasted. A close relative reports successful treatment with ultrasound for a bruise that did not go away after treatment with external hot packs and local massage. Such modalities, now commonly used by dancers and athletes, are available only under close supervision of a physician.

PREPARING YOURSELF TO FIGHT PAIN

☐ At first inkling that you may develop a persistent pain, "throw heat" at it immediately, or use any other modality recommended to fight it. The earlier you catch it and eliminate it, the more time you save in the long run. Hot packs, hot-water soaks, whirlpool baths usually take twenty minutes to a half-hour, and while you may resent the time involved, these measures have to be taken for therapeutic reasons. "Working off" a pain that has settled down may take many months, as I experienced with my neck, jaw, back, and shoulders.

Be sure you have on hand whatever aids you need to immobilize a joint. These would include Ace bandages for painful ankles, elbows, or knees. I have observed that I can eliminate the hurt in an ankle by wrapping it overnight in an Ace bandage. Failing to do this could mean pain persisting throughout the next day indicating additional irritational damage, which will then take longer to remedy.

Hand-rest splints should always be kept available to be used immediately, when necessary.

Note: For information about how you can obtain the devices and special equipment mentioned in this chapter, consult the Directory of Aids.

Some Aids to Optimum Health and Comfort 5

☐ For arthritics, it is not so easy to keep smiling. Pain and disability make this difficult, to say the least, so we should not overlook any of the available ways to make life easier.

In addition to the various treatment modalities I have already discussed, there are other important aspects of care that can ease the experience of living with arthritis. Among those I discuss here are sleep, nutrition, climate, and visits to special treatment centers.

CREATING CONDITIONS FOR SOUND SLEEP

☐ We normally sleep for about eight hours, which means that we spend one-third of our time in bed. For arthritics, this time may easily be ten or twelve hours, including rest periods during the day. This means that we arthritics spend nearly half our lives in bed. So we might as well be comfortable while we sleep. If we are poorly supported, this may have bad effects on our posture, breathing, and circulation during the day. A defectively designed sleeping support can act like an ill-fitting splint, which, when worn for a long period, can add to deformity and be detrimental to our health.

Sleep is supposed to rest the body as completely as possible. During this rest period, the heart beats at a slower pace, since the requirements on circulation are reduced. It is important for the heart to be able to rest in this way, in order to meet the increased demands of the next day. (I owe this interpretation to Dr. Christiaan Barnard, the pioneer heart surgeon. He discussed a novel heart operation in which he planned to disconnect the impaired heart of a patient and use the heart of a donor or a chimpanzee to temporarily operate the patient's circulatory system. The object of this procedure was to let the patient's heart recover during a period of total rest. Eventually, the recovered heart would be reconnected and the auxiliary heart disconnected.)

Every night, we rest our heart by permitting our pulse rate to drop from, say, eighty to ninety beats per minute at full activity, down to perhaps sixty beats per minute or less at full nighttime rest. Simultaneously, the body temperature drops somewhat, because our muscles, which generate most of the heat to sustain body temperature, are now largely inactive.

BLANKETS

☐ The matter of body temperature brings us to the first sleep-comfort requirement: a proper cover. If we lie down to sleep uncovered, we will feel chilly in the same temperature that felt comfortable when we were up and moving. This is because the muscles are not working to supply heat. If we are chilled enough, we will start to shiver, which is a natural defensive reflex to generate heat in the muscles. So in winter be sure you keep yourself warm. An electric blanket is both lightweight and uniformly warm. (The latest models are generally rated as completely safe.) In summer you can substitute a regular or thermal blanket.

PILLOWS

☐ The matter of pillows is not quite so simple. I analyzed the function of various pillows as they would influence my body and sleeping comfort, in order to come to the best solution myself, and will summarize my findings for you here. I realize that your needs may not be identical to mine, but you may learn something from my analysis.

Sleeping comfort—or discomfort—is obtained in any of these possible sleeping positions: lying on your (1) back, (2) side, and (3) stomach. Furthermore, we have to judge our sleeping arrangements on how well they satisfy the requirements of (1) the skeletal system and (2) the circulatory system.

From a skeletal point of view, it is probably best to use a small pillow, or a thin, soft pillow, or no pillow at all, when you are lying on your back. In this posture the upper spinal column is straight and there is less danger of compression on the roots of the nerves that emanate from the spinal cord. The muscles are relaxed and there is little strain on ligaments. With a soft pillow, the head sinks in deeply, and the neck is held fairly straight. When you roll on your side, the pillow helps keep the upper spinal column properly aligned (figs. 1 and 2). For sleeping or resting on your side, use whatever pillow arrangement you like to keep the neck comfortably aligned with the rest of the spinal column.

When you sleep on your side, a thin pillow, or a small ear pillow (what the French call an *oreiller*) will help to keep the neck properly aligned.

From the point of view of the circulatory system, it is preferable to sleep with the upper part of the body slightly propped up, since this places less strain on the heart. I can attest to this. At times, when I had a heart problem, I awoke in the middle of the night

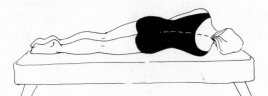

1. *Neck forms angle with spine; uncomfortable*

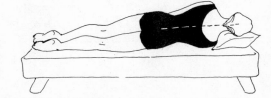

2. *Thin pillow straightens out neck and spine*

gasping for air. Sleeping with the upper part of my body propped up and the windows open gave immediate and dramatic relief. My doctor explained that when one lies flat the heart has to work harder to avoid accumulation of fluids in the upper torso. Less work is needed when the force of gravity aids in draining fluids away from the upper torso. I think we can infer from this that even normal individuals can benefit from sleeping with the upper torso raised. The obvious way to accomplish this is to sleep with two or three pillows elevating the shoulders and head. There is a disadvantage to this arrangement, however, in that the shoulders then tend to become rounded when you sleep on your back, and this is not an optimal position for expansion of your chest cavity to permit proper breathing. However, you can have both a raised position and unrestricted breathing by using a wedge of the sort that is popular in certain countries of northern Europe. This is a firm, wedge-shaped pillow, of a consistency similar to the mattress, made, for instance, of foam rubber, which elevates the upper torso and head and allows the shoulders to lie flat. This really is a most comfortable arrangement. All you need when you roll over to the side is a thin pillow to support your head, unless you require also some support of your head when lying on your back. (I have described a combination of three small baby pillows for this purpose in chapter 6.)

For the lower torso and legs, we want a position in which there is little or no muscular activity and as little stress as possible on the joints, to prevent unconscious shifting of position, which could cause pain and wake us up. Especially if we have lower back problems, we want the position of greatest relaxation for the trunk and legs. Authors who have analyzed back problems recommend the fetal position during sleep. This is the position the fetus assumes in the womb (fig. 3). The lower back is straight, the upper back and head are curled, and the knees are brought toward

3. *Pillow helps with the fetal position*

the chest. In this posture, too, we tend to keep the mouth closed, and so avoid the dry mouth and snoring that can wake us up when we sleep on our back.

THE BED

☐ All would be ideal if beds were designed for greatest comfort, but this is far from the current reality. Perhaps it is just not possible to design a bed that is comfortable in both sleeping positions—on your back and on your side. The most popular design today is the very firm mattress for "firm support to the lower back." A very firm mattress (or one with a bedboard underneath) allows you to roll easily onto your side. A soft mattress, especially one that sags in the middle, requires quite some effort from your back muscles as you roll over onto your side, which can cause you to wrench your back and so wake you up. When you roll over onto your side on a firm mattress, your back feels comfortable, but the hard contact between the mattress and your shoulder and hips eventually becomes uncomfortable, and so you roll over onto your back again. However, you may not be comfortable on your back, since the lower back tends to become hollow in this posture unless you put a pillow under your knees.

All the above analysis is intended to show how difficult it is to arrive at the most comfortable bed and sleeping arrangements. I have actually been quite comfortable and relaxed in a rope hammock, the type with a wooden bar at the head end, which permits the shoulders to be extended. I could sleep in the hammock for several hours without waking up. The netting conforms to the body without undue localized pressure and permits the lower back to be straight. The trouble is that eventually you want to move your legs to increase lymph and venous circulation, and that is difficult to do in a hammock. Also, getting into and out of a hammock can be a problem for some arthritics.

Here is the combination I have arrived at for promoting comfort in all positions. I use a high-resilience, high-compression, firm, four-inch foam-rubber mattress, topped by a two-inch, medium-to-soft foam-rubber mattress cover. I place these on a box spring with a wooden bedboard in between the mattress and the box spring. The two-inch mattress cover supplies sufficient softness of contact for my hips and shoulders when I roll over to the side; it also permits the buttocks to sink in slightly, allowing the lower back to assume a proper contour. I do occasionally use a pillow under my knees when my back problem flares up. (The pillow under the knees is not generally advised for arthritics, since it promotes hip flexion, which can eventually result in flexion contraction of the hip.)

A frequent piece of advice to arthritics is to lie on the stomach for at least half an hour a day to keep the hip flexors extended and prevent them from contracting. After ten years of rheumatoid arthritis, I found it quite difficult to roll onto my stomach, and more so to roll back again. Shoulder, arm, and back muscles had to be strained considerably, and eventually they could not accomplish the job. However, as long as you can roll onto your stomach, it is probably good to do this at least once a day. In this position, you do not want to use the wedge pillow; instead support your head with a thin, small pillow when you turn your head to the side.

YOUR SUPPLY OF FRESH AIR

☐ A few words about the air we breathe during our sleep. We want as much breathing comfort as possible so that we will not awake in discomfort or put unnecessary strain on our heart. The optimum conditions may be different for different people. For some, a very low humidity may cause a dry, parched throat. With too much humidity, perspiration cannot evaporate from your skin and you may become sweaty. All this should influence whether or not you sleep with the window open. I avoid opening the window at night when the atmospheric conditions outside are particularly disagreeable; on the other hand, a slightly opened window allows negative ions (atoms charged with negative electricity) to come in freely from the outdoors, producing in us the feeling of breathing fresh air. This effect is exaggerated in the mountains or near a waterfall, where there are plenty of negative ions in the air. (To my knowledge, no complete explanation is available for this effect.)

You may have wondered about the usefulness of electronic "air fresheners." These units, which are high-voltage generators, carry small antennae which emit negative ions or attract positive ions. The ions in the air tend to precipitate odor-producing bacteria, as well as other kinds of small particles, such as dust, bacteria, and pollen, to the ground. As a result, the air actually is cleansed and feels fresh. Industrially, where air cleaning is necessary to remove all dust from the air, as in film processing, large machines called precipitrons are installed which precipitate dust particles so that they do not come in contact with the materials to be kept clean. I mention this to encourage your trust in the small home units. Skepticism is understandable, since the action of the air fresheners is invisible and can't be "smelled" immediately, as can chemical air fresheners.

Some years ago, so-called germicidal lamps were introduced for use in the kitchen. These have a similar effect in precipitating or "killing" bacteria, and the "fresh air" can be smelled as ozone is produced; this is the smell you sometimes observe in nature after lightning. The drawback here is that ozone is unhealthy if inhaled for extended periods.

The most comfortable ambient air temperature for humans is between 65° and 75° F (18°–23° C). At night, one usually prefers a temperature closer to the lower rather than the upper limit, provided there is adequate covering.

ADJUSTING TO CHANGES OF TEMPERATURE

☐ Elsewhere I have mentioned the importance of covering vulnerable joints to protect them from becoming chilled. It is just as important in arthritis to keep the *entire* body comfortably clothed for the conditions of climate and temperature you are in. Since becoming an arthritic, I find I have difficulty in maintaining a uniform temperature on the surface of my body. When the cold season approaches, I feel easily chilled and my joints start to hurt. It has been reported that arthritics suffer more during a change of climate than during a uniformly cool climate. (This completely corresponds to my experience.) However, during cool weather, there are considerable temperature variations between outdoors and indoors, and the body is stressed by having to adjust to these changes. Certain choices of clothing can help you make these temperature transitions with a minimum of stress. Particularly helpful in the chilly season is a type of thin, woollen underwear manufactured in Europe. I was able to locate this in better department stores . I find that it keeps me warm but not so warm to induce perspiration. Also available from Europe are protective body-warmers for practically every joint of the body (See Directory of Aids. See also figure 42, page 270).

So the rule for clothing in chilly weather is two-part:

1. Avoid getting chilled (and if you get even the slightest twinge resulting from a chill, take steps to alleviate it with heat, bandages, warm underwear, or other means).
2. Avoid overdressing to the point where you start to perspire; a draft hitting a perspired area is likely to result in muscle spasm, which will not go away easily by itself.

From the remarks about clothing, it may be inferred that a uniformly mild, warm climate is most comfortable for arthritics. There is one condition, however: it should be a dry rather than a humid climate. Humidity presents a considerable stress on the temperature regulating mechanism of our bodies, since a good percentage of the temperature regulation is accomplished by evaporation of water from the skin, and this is considerably inhibited by external humidity. Notice that furry animals suffer greatly during hot, humid weather. The panting that dogs do in such weather is an attempt to rid themselves of excess body heat by evaporation from their tongues.

Overly warm and humid climates may require air conditioning, which again, produces stressful temperature differentials between indoors and outdoors. The most pleasant temperature range is from 65° to 75° F (18°–23° C) with low to medium humidity. At low humidity, the nights can be expected to be cool. An electric blanket is especially helpful then because it is so easily adjustable.

HOW'S YOUR DIET?

□ The subject of nutrition in arthritis is somewhat controversial. Books have been written promising cures through diet, but the medical establishment tends to ignore this approach. All the physicians I have spoken to, however, do stress the importance of a "healthy" diet. By this they mean eating lots of fruits and vegetables, keeping intake of proteins and carbohydrates in good balance (a ratio of about one to six respectively), and passing up junk food—the overprocessed, overrefined, oversweetened, highly caloric, and nutrient-poor foods that form so large a part of the American diet. The vegetables and fruit are especially important for rheumatoid arthritis sufferers, who need iron to keep their hemoglobin count up to favorable levels. Iron is available in all green vegetables and in many fruits. (Iron supplements tend to produce constipation, and thus the natural sources are preferable.)

As far as vitamin supplements are concerned, various doctors, including my rheumatologist, Dr. Otto Steinbrocker, have recommended daily use of vitamin C. This vitamin, too, has been the subject of controversy. Quite apart from the unproven claims made for it, it is indeed important. It is necessary for the utilization of iron, and it is known to be helpful in cell repair. Many people believe that it can prevent colds. I have been able to stop a cold in the early stages by using recommended amounts of vitamin C, at least one gram per day. I consider vitamin C a food supplement rather than a medication. I am fully aware that it may not give everybody the same advantage; indeed, I am unable to say whether the benefits I have gotten are physiologically or mentally induced (the so-called placebo effect). But I do not dispute the known beneficial properties of vitamin C, which cause so many physicians to recommend it.

VACATIONS CAN HELP YOU COPE

☐ One of the unfortunate consequences of arthritis is the keen sense we have of being prevented from doing so many things we want to do. At times we may feel depressed and it takes strong efforts to throw off this feeling. We put ourselves in the best position to remain active by doing our exercises—doing them daily so that we can derive their cumulative benefits, and doing them within an allotted, brief time so that we don't let the management of our disease push work as well as leisure activities out of our lives.

For some of my readers, it may also be possible to take an occasional vacation especially geared to helping you get relief from the discomforts of arthritis. I would encourage any such plan, provided you make careful inquiries about the facilities before you go. I have been to several of these vacation spots and have found the European facilities on the whole both more pleasant and more beneficial than those currently available in the United States.

If you have never been to a European spa, the following brief account of a visit I made to Monte Grotto, in Italy, may be of interest.

The setting of the Garden hotel in Monte Grotto provides guests with a view of rolling hills and luxurious gardens. The rooms and baths are exquisitely appointed. You can enjoy breakfast on your balcony.

Both midday and evening meals offer many courses and a large variety of choices. Fresh fruit and vegetables are abundant, fresh cuts of meats and fresh fish are always available, and special diets can be accommodated. It is even possible to have your meal at poolside. I mention these details just to show that such a spa furnishes, in addition to treatment, the perfect relaxation of a vacation. The visitors, mostly from northern Europe, come to Monte Grotto to treat their twinges of arthritis in the warm water and take the prophylactic mud treatment. The usual stay is three weeks. The outdoor swimming pool has a pleasant temperature just below body temperature, which relaxes the muscles and permits them to be stretched to the maximum.

I arrived in Monte Grotto with extremely painful shoulders and upper back which prevented me from sleeping properly at night. Earlier I had tried tissue massage and hot-pack treatments, which helped somewhat as long as I carried on the treatment. Cortisone shots into the shoulders had given only temporary relief. I therefore came to Monte Grotto with great expectations.

Within one hour of our arrival I was looked over by a physician in my hotel room. He checked my heart to find out whether I could stand the strain of the muscle treatment and decided I could do it without any heart stimulant (although he prescribed this for me during my treatment in the third year).

My first treatment was at seven o'clock the following morning. I was guided to the basement via elevator by an adorable little boy, who escorted me both to the treatment and back. In the treatment room there was a cot onto which about one pailful of steaming mud (*fango*) was spread out by the attendant. I was asked to lie down on this cot and found it painfully hot for a few seconds. The attendant then proceeded to take steaming mud from other pails and apply it to my body, until I was entirely enveloped in hot mud, with the exception of my head. I could not move at all in this hot mud pie. I remained in this condition under the watchful eye of the attendant for twenty minutes. My little guide remained also in the room and applied cold compresses to my forehead, renewing them once in a while. After twenty minutes, I was asked to get up and shed my armor of mud. I was rinsed clean by a hot spray from the nozzle of a garden hose aimed at me by the attendant. Next I was asked to step down into a kind of Roman bath filled with hot water from the Monte Grotto spring. It was permeated with bubbles of ozone and felt pleasant and prickly on the body. After fifteen minutes of this I was helped out of the bath, dried, clothed in my bathrobe, and taken back up to my room by my little guide. This time I could really use him, since the treatment had left me quite weak. I rested on the bed still wrapped in my bathrobe, with which I was still wisely covered to absorb the ensuing perspiration. I was warned beforehand that I would perspire, and this was an important part of the treatment. I felt very relaxed and often fell asleep during this time.

Next a masseur arrived, who gave me a very gentle, very rapid surface massage (*effleurage*). He massaged away from the joints, never touching the joints themselves, and he did not knead the muscles. It was just a rapid, gentle stroking. During the massage he administered passive motion exercises to various joints—my first experience of passive exercising in four to five years of arthritis. I realized then how restricted my shoulder movements had become. I cannot say for sure whether the masseur succeeded in increasing the range of motion of my shoulders, but I can definitely state that the pain in my shoulders was reduced after several weeks of this treatment, so that I could easily roll onto my shoulders at night without being awakened by pain.

(I have described this treatment in some detail because such descriptions are seldom found in the brochures sent out by spas. Usually they show a picture of a person fully enveloped in mud, but I think that an

American reader wants to know more about what he is getting himself into.)

After the massage you may breakfast in bed or on your balcony, then enjoy the rest of the day just as you would in any vacation resort, with sightseeing and entertainment. You may go for an afternoon swim in the thermal pool, or if the weather is poor, enjoy a somewhat warmer indoor pool. The mud treatment in the morning and the afternoon swim in the warm water were not a strain for me, but rather a great relaxation.

After this first visit to Monte Grotto my shoulders remained pain-free for about half a year, until the beginning of winter. I then resumed hot-pack treatments and massages in New York with results that fell far short of the experience in Monte Grotto, but I managed better than the year before. I visited Monte Grotto twice more in the following years, with ever longer-lasting relief in my shoulders. Since the third visit to Monte Grotto, ten years ago, I have never had the same shoulder pain again. My range of motion of the shoulders remains somewhat limited, however, and although I recovered some of my strength in the arms that was lost in the years of pain and nonuse I cannot say that this recovery was complete. It is clear to me that proper exercises in the first few years of the disease would have preserved more range of motion. It is possible that maintaining that range of motion would have permitted me to "work away" the pain, using heat, exercise, and massage, and the newer modality of ultrasound, which was not available to me at that time. Unfortunately, I must say that three years of treatment in Monte Grotto did not prevent pain and damage in other joints. I cannot predict if I would have been helped by going to Monte Grotto every year.

A few years ago I visited the spa in Switzerland called Bad Ragaz. The Hotel Hof Ragaz, which is connected to the bathhouse by a corridor, is a luxury hotel of the first order, with cuisine that cannot be surpassed. Neither can the prices. Fortunately, there are more reasonably priced hotels in the town, although then one has to walk through the streets to reach the bathhouse, which may be somewhat risky in rainy weather.

The bath facilities are two very large warm pools at slightly different temperatures, just under body temperature. There are strong jets of water along the edges of the pools, at various heights of the body, so that when you walk along the inside perimeter of a pool holding onto the rail, your knees, your hips, and shoulders are sprayed.

In addition to the pools, a superb medical and physical set-up is available. Medical specialists for rheumatology, heart and orthopedic surgery, as well as physical medicine, are in attendance. I was prescribed underwater exercise sessions, which were carried out in a small private pool with an excellent therapist who taught me the importance of the small muscle groups of the hips, knees, and ankles to help maintain equilibrium when standing. I also had daily physical therapy sessions which enlarged my knowledge about exercises for feet, ankles, and toes.

I firmly believe that a spa in the United States incorporating the best aspects of Monte Grotto and Bad Ragaz would be a great success and would provide a valuable service to arthritic patients. If it were staffed by physical therapists and medical personnel, some reimbursement from Medicare and similar plans might be feasible. It could provide valuable electronic treatment methods, such as ultrasound, and also massage. Massage following a heat application is very helpful in relaxing the muscles and reducing pain, but unfortunately, as a home treatment, massage is quite expensive.

The Europeans are enjoying valuable hydrotherapy treatment during the early stages of the disease as a prophylactic method. I believe that we deserve this in the United States too.

It may be useful to explain the words *spa* and *cure* as they are used in Europe. We associate the word *spa* with famous mineral-spring resorts such as Saratoga in New York State, or Marienbad in Czechoslovakia. The spas I have mentioned have nothing to do with "drinking the waters." Nor should you understand the word *cure* as meaning a cure for arthritis. The German word *Kur* and the Italian word *cura* refer merely to the place in the town or village where the treatment takes place. The *Kuranstalt* is the establishment where the waters are dispensed to people seeking relief for digestive ailments, and for other places where hydrotherapy is available.

Part 2

CONTAINS DETAILED instructions for the all-important five-minute daily tense-relax-and-stretch routine (this chapter comes last for ready reference), as well as detailed exercises for stretching and strengthening various parts of the body.

Each chapter stands on its own. If, for example, you are particularly interested in exercises for the hands, you may go directly to the relevant chapter and concentrate your efforts on that part of the body.

Plan to spend five to fifteen minutes on each category of exercise. The durations I suggest are: for the neck and jaws, five minutes; for the shoulders and elbows, ten minutes; for posture, breathing, and circulation, five to ten minutes; for hips, lower back, and knees, fifteen minutes; for the feet and ankles, five minutes. Don't be discouraged if it takes you longer to do the exercises the first time around; you will pick up speed with practice.

The various categories of exercise can be done on successive nights of the week, as the titles of the chapters indicate. Any sequence that suits you will do, however, so long as you do the exercises regularly.

To get maximum results from the daily five-minute tense-relax-and-stretch routine, you should be well acquainted with the materials in the other exercise chapters.

THE CHAPTERS

Monday Night: Neck and Jaw

6

Testing the ranges of neck motion, figures 1–6

□ Most of us have experienced a stiff neck at one time or another in our lives, and often after the stiff neck is gone there is some residual discomfort. Whether or not you are arthritic—and you need not consider yourself so just because you have a stiff neck—it is desirable to keep the neck as flexible as possible, since a stiff neck can cause sleepless nights and headaches. After trying massages, heat, and traction with only temporary relief, I found the following exercises to be pain-free and dramatically effective. As with all exercises, if you are in treatment with a physician, get his approval before you begin.

1. Bend head all the way to the right.

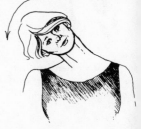

TESTING THE NECK RANGES

□ Before you start exercising, make the following test to find out if your neck is sufficiently flexible or if it needs improvement.

2. Now all the way to the left, ear close to shoulder.

• Sit on a chair in front of a mirror and lower the head to one side as far as possible. It should come close to the shoulder without your having to raise the shoulder (fig. 1). Do the same motion to the other side (fig. 2). If you are able to move your head in this way—

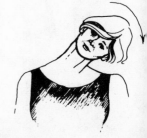

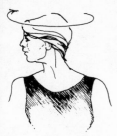

3. *Turn head to right to look over your shoulder.*

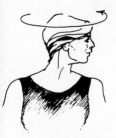

4. *Rotate head to the opposite side.*

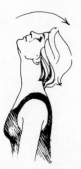

5. *Move head all the way back, so that the nape touches the back.*

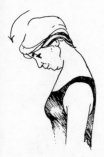

6. *Now all the way forward, so that chin touches chest.*

almost touching either shoulder—without pain, then you have what is called full range of motion. If you cannot do this, your range is limited.

Even if the range of motion is not severely limited, it is advisable to obtain as broad a range as possible, although the side motion of the head is not used much in daily activity. An example of its use might be a traveler who drops off to sleep on a long plane ride and lets his head fall to one side: he may wake with pain from the abnormal pull of the muscles of the cervical spine (the seven vertebrae that make up the neck) if he has restricted range of motion.

• The next test for flexibility is to rotate the head first to one side (fig. 3) and then to the other (fig. 4). You have sufficient range of motion if you can rotate the head without difficulty so that the nose is almost in line with the shoulders and you can look slightly behind you.

This range of motion is important in daily life; for example, when you drive a car and turn your head back to check traffic, you should not feel pain.

• The final check for flexibility is to move your head all the way back (fig. 5), and all the way forward (fig. 6). You have sufficient range if the back of your head touches the nape of your neck, and in the forward position if the chin touches the chest.

Most people can touch the chin to the chest, since this motion occurs in many of our daily activities as we observe what we are doing with our hands—in typing, cooking, eating, and so forth. The backward movement (as in gargling) is rarely used, so there is a tendency for tension and stiffness to develop.

Stiffness that inhibits motion causes metabolic products to accumulate in the tense muscles, and pain can result. This could be: (1) local pain within the muscle itself, (2) sharp twinges of nerve pain due to imbalanced muscle pull around the cervical spine, and/or (3) headaches caused by poor circulation in the neck.

My intention here is not to help you diagnose your condition, but to illustrate conditions in which exercise can be beneficial. Arthritic pain in any part of the body, especially the lower part of the body (feet, knees, hips), very often results in tightening of the neck muscles. Mental tension can have the same effect, causing pain and a decrease in the range of motion.

EXERCISING THE NECK RANGES

☐ We now come to the exercises. After telling you how to do them I will discuss my own experience in doing them and the benefits I have received.

Exercising the neck ranges, sideways bending of head, figures 7a–12

Bending Sideways

• Sit on a chair in front of the mirror, and as a starting position for the exercise, pull the chin in, push the neck back, and raise the head straight up (figs. 7a, 7b). Be as relaxed as possible in doing this; remem-

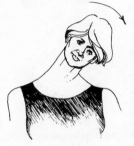

8. *Bend head to left as far as it will go.*

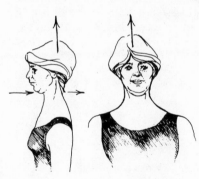

7a & 7b. *Pull chin in, push back of neck out, raise head up.*

ber this is only the starting position of the exercise itself. If you have great difficulty in obtaining the starting position, practice it for ten seconds a few times daily.

Bend head down with left ear toward left shoulder —*gently* (fig. 8). Observe in the mirror where you come to a stop. To avoid pain, don't go beyond that point.

At the point where you stopped, place your right hand against your right temple and press your head against your hand as firmly as possible (fig. 9). Hold for two to three seconds (count of six). Now relax for a second or two. Next, move your head gently lower down. Unless you were able almost to bring your ear close to your shoulder in the first place, you will notice you can lower your head a little more (fig. 10). Repeat the exercise as long as you continue to gain range (ear closer to shoulder).

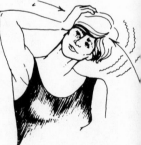

9. *Press temple hard against hand, count to six, relax.*

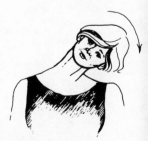

10. *Try gently to lower head further down toward left shoulder.*

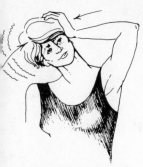

11. *Press your left temple against your left hand, firmly for the count of six, relax.*

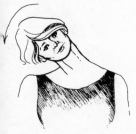

12. *Gently lower head farther toward right side.*

Complementary Exercise

• Repeat the same exercise for the other side. Place the left hand to the left temple, bending the head down with the right ear toward the right shoulder— gently (fig. 11). Observe in the mirror where you come to a stop. To avoid pain, don't go beyond that point. Press head firmly against left hand to count of six. Relax. Gently lower head farther toward the right shoulder (fig. 12).

Rotations

• From the same starting position—namely, with your chin in, neck back, head up (fig. 13)—rotate your head toward your left shoulder until you come to a stop (fig. 14). Rotate as far as you can without experiencing pain. At this point, place your right hand on your right temple and rotate your head firmly backward against the hand in the opposite direction with-

Head rotation exercises, figures 13–18

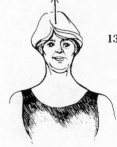

13. *Starting position*

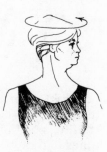

14. *Rotate head to left until you come to a stop.*

out permitting the hand to move (fig. 15). Hold for two to three seconds (count of six). Relax for a second or two and rotate the head again in the direction of the left shoulder as far as possible. You will notice in the mirror that you have gained a little more motion (fig. 16). If your range was very restricted, you may

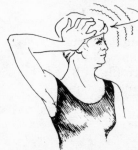

15. *Press head firmly against hand for a count of six, relax.*

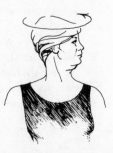

16. *Rotate head further, as far as you can.*

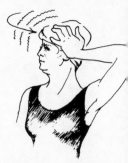

repeat the exercise by pressing against your hand, relaxing, and rotating further. This may be repeated two or three times until you find that you are not increasing range.

Complementary Exercise

• Now repeat the same exercise for the other side. Place your left hand on the left temple and rotate the head toward the right shoulder. Observe in the mirror where you come to a stop. To avoid pain, don't go beyond this point. Rotate your head firmly backward against the hand without permitting the hand to move (fig. 17). Hold for two to three seconds. Relax for a second or two and rotate the head again in the direction of the right shoulder (fig. 18). Repeat a few times if you notice that you are still gaining range.

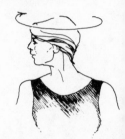

17. *Press head firmly against hand count of six, relax.*

18. *Rotate head toward right shoulder as far as you can.*

Bending Backward and Forward

• From a standing position with the neck straight (fig. 19), move the head gently backward as far as you can without discomfort, and stop there (fig. 20). Place both hands against the forehead and press the head firmly against the hands for two to three seconds (count of six) without permitting the hands to move (fig. 21). Relax for a second or two. Now move the head gently farther back (fig. 22). You will probably

Bending head backward and forward, figures 19–25

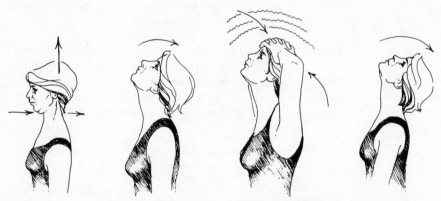

19. *Starting position*

20. *Bend head back as far as it will go.*

21. *Press head firmly against hands for a count of six, relax.*

22. *Move farther back if you can.*

feel that you gained a little more range, unless you were able to touch the nape of your neck with your head in the first place.

You may repeat, pressing forward against your hands and then moving the head further back, as long as you can feel you can increase the range somewhat. Don't repeat the exercise more than two or three times each session. Instead, have a few sessions each day, especially if you are starting out with a very limited range.

• Move head gently forward and down until you come to a stop (fig. 23). If your chin does not quite touch your chest, you have less than full range of motion. Hold both hands in back of your head. Push your head back firmly against your hands, without letting your hands move, for two to three seconds (count of six) (fig. 24). Relax for a second or two then move the head farther forward and down, trying to touch your chest with your chin (fig. 25). Most people can reach this quickly with the first or second attempt.

I call the three preceding exercises tense-relax-and-stretch exercises. (They use the technique of proprioceptive neuromuscular facilitation [PNF] which I describe in chapter 3.) Here is an additional (optional) exercise: rolling your head in as wide a circle as possible. I believe it has usefulness for checking your range of motion in all angles. From a biomechanical point of view, this exercise does not include the relaxation that would make it efficient for gaining additional range. However, it follows the tried principle of PNF, in that you move from a pain-free range into a more limited range that normally would produce pain.

• Describe the biggest possible circle you can with the tip of your nose. Starting with the position in Fig. 26a, rotate your head as shown.
• *Complementary Exercise:* Repeat this exercise by rotating the head in the opposite direction (fig. 26b).

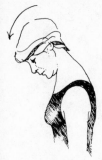

23. *Move head forward until you come to a stop.*

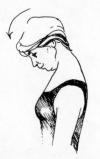

24. *Push head firmly back against hands for a count of six, relax.*

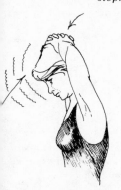

25. *Bend farther down to touch chin to chest.*

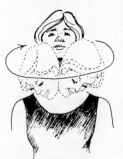

26a. *Rotate head to describe the biggest possible circle with your nose.*

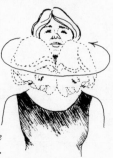

26b. *Repeat in the opposite direction.*

RELIEF FROM NECK PAIN

☐ It may be helpful to you to hear about my experiences with neck problems and how the above exercises worked for me, as compared to other types of therapies such as heat and massage. Neck problems are not a typical rheumatoid arthritic condition of the sort represented by an inflamed, swollen, and painful joint. The neck consists of a number of vertebrae which are able to move against each other in various directions, thereby facilitating flexion. In my case the decrease of range started very early during my first strong attack of arthritis. I developed an acute sensitivity to drafts and experienced such strong spasms in some of the muscles at the back of the head that even a small motion of the head caused me excruciating pain. I obtained some relief by using hot compresses, wearing a warm scarf, and avoiding drafts, but I don't believe I could have done any of the exercises described above without sharp pain.

Twelve years after the first attack, I developed a different type of involvement, which I would call a stiff neck. I first noticed it when I began feeling uncomfortable sleeping with two pillows. I tried changing to one pillow and finally sleeping with no pillow, but I still could not get comfortable when lying down. My rheumatologist applied head traction a number of times in his office, each time for about five minutes, with increasing weights. This felt extremely comfortable and gave me some respite from neck pain. By that time spring had arrived, which may have helped to increase my overall flexibility.

When the next winter came along, the neck condition started up again and became much worse. I had pain not only when lying down but with every slight movement of the head. My physician then prescribed a traction device for daily home use. I also applied hot compresses. When all this did not help I was prescribed a soft collar. This orthopedic device is worn around the neck during the day or night, or both, to immobilize the neck and thereby to relax the muscles and relieve pain. The collar—first a soft and later a hard collar—proved quite comfortable while I wore it but pain returned when I removed it. For sleeping, I was told to use an air pillow and to blow it up to the point where my neck felt comfortable. This was not very successful, however. Finally, after nearly a year, X-rays of the neck were taken which showed some osteoarthritic deposits. These deposits reduced the size of the openings in the vertebrae (the foramina) through which the nerves pass. One physician thought this might account for the pain. There seemed to be no rheumatoid change in the cervical spine.

Physicians had told me all along that exercise was essential, but they had given me very little actual instruction. To increase the range, I was told to push my head, at first gently and then more firmly, against the limit of the existing range. "Move your head from side to side three to ten times, and every time you come to the end of the range give it a little push." I found this quite painful and saw little sense in taking painkillers and applying local heat merely in order to do these exercises.

I finally researched the literature of the subject and found in Cailliet's *Neck and Arm Pain* a reference to the "Rhythmic Stabilization Technique" used for loosening neck muscles (see Bibliography). Here the patient does isometric contractions by leaning the head against the resisting hands of the therapist. I have come across a similar technique called "Hold, Relax" by Voss (see Bibliography, authors Knott and Voss), and I remembered that a therapist a few years earlier had used this type of exercise to extend the range of my shoulder. I adapted all these techniques to the motions usually recommended for the neck—namely, bending sideways, rotating sideways, bending forward and backward. Note that by *stretch* I mean stretching the muscles, not the tissue of the neck, which could be painful.

Another possible factor in muscle pain is the presence of metabolic products such as lactic acid. If not removed quickly enough from the muscle, these products may cause irritation. In order to remove these products efficiently, the muscle has to function properly; blood must be pumped regularly through the muscle in order to flush away the metabolic products. But this is not possible so long as the muscle is in a spastic and painful condition. The muscle first has to be relaxed.

When there is pain, a sort of vicious cycle starts, since the pain produces a "protective spasm" in the muscles—that is, a reflex reaction to the pain in the form of a forceful muscle contraction. Traction removes pain by easing pressure between the tightly packed vertebrae. Release of pain also releases much of the protective spasm. This is probably why, at the start of my neck condition, the temporary release of spasm during traction was sufficient to get the muscle operating properly and to remove the metabolic toxins.

Toxic substances within the muscle are not to be thought of as serious poisons. They are normal products of muscle activity. But if they are not regularly removed, they tend to irritate the muscle and produce pain. After a vigorous workout or a performance, an athlete has a large amount of toxicity in his muscles and may appear quite stiff and uncomfortable. That is why a hot shower, massage, and gentle exercise are usually routine treatment after sports.

I mention all this because when I became arthritic I experienced a stiffness and pain very similar to what the athlete feels. The great difference is that as one gets older it is not as easy to get rid of these aches and pains. But the physical means both for prevention and treatment are in many ways similar. When I had my first neck involvement and found relief in wearing a warm scarf and avoiding drafts, I was reminded of the boxer who generally puts a towel around his neck when leaving the ring. After a workout the body is very hot and the neck is susceptible to drafts; the towel affords protection. The arthritic does not have to go through this heating and cooling process to be susceptible to drafts, especially during the winter months.

I obtained considerable relief after I started working alone on the neck exercises I had researched. After doing them for a few days, I was so enthusiastic about the increase in range—actually seeing it in the mirror —that I did the exercises two or three times a day. At the same time, I was also able to adapt better to the so-called cervical pillow, a long bolster of about six inches in diameter, which I had not been able to use before. After about one month of daily exercise and using the cervical pillow, I could "forget about" my neck.

PILLOWS FOR NECK COMFORT

□ Cervical pillows come in various sizes and types to suit individual needs. An air pillow can be blown up to the thickness that raises the head to the most comfort-

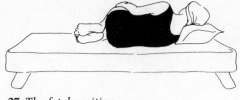

27. *The fetal position*

able level for the user. The bolster-type pillow is available in several different diameters. In addition, there are pillows with a contoured cutout for the head. Pillows of this type are available in various thicknesses, firmnesses, and cutout sizes from surgical supply stores. I tried several sizes and could not find comfort with any of them. Someone with an acute neck condition may have the same experience.

I found that after lying still on my back for any length of time I developed pain in my neck and needed to turn over onto one side, then later onto the other side (tossing and turning). There is one other design of cervical pillow which theoretically could provide comfort in just this case. It is made with a soft filling, and while one is lying on one's side the spine is held in a straight line all the way, preventing a sharp angle at the base of the neck. This is an excellent idea. However, I found it necessary to make my own thicker version of this arrangement, one that would also support me in the fetal position (head forward, knees up, as in figure 27). In order to be able to slide my head forward and be supported in this position, I had three baby pillows sewn together, as shown in figure 28.

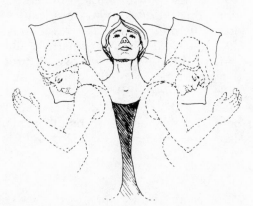

28. *Three baby pillows stitched together as shown. Your neck is supported when you are on your back as well as curled up on your side.*

The pillow in the middle supports the neck, and the pillows on either side support the head when one is resting on one's side, in the fetal position. The pillows may be sewn together. I found this arrangement extremely confortable. It can be easily adjusted by choosing different thicknesses for the various pillows. I have described this arrangement in some detail so the reader can construct his or her own combination, since this type of pillow so far is not available commercially. I also described this in detail to underline the fact that exercising the neck is not enough; you must try to keep a very relaxed position during sleep. If you do not, the neck becomes more spastic all the time, and you are deprived of the benefits of a good night's rest. (See chapter 5 for more information on sleep comfort.) It is entirely possible that the neck condition will improve by itself if the neck is sufficiently relaxed during the night and is permitted to move normally during daily activities. This might get rid of toxins so that no further deliberate exercises are necessary. However, the deliberate exercises are useful for rapidly increasing range of motion and for achieving a more upright neck position.

SUGGESTED FREQUENCY AND DURATION OF EXERCISES

□ It seems to me, from what I have observed and from my own experience, that arthritics, or people with back trouble or neck trouble, do exercises only as a last resort, when they are suffering very much and can no longer be helped by painkillers. This is very sad, since an ounce of prevention in these cases is worth more than ten pounds of cure. Once a back or neck condition, or any other joint condition, has settled in, it takes a concentrated effort to relieve it, and complete relief may be impossible. Daily motion exercises to maintain and improve flexibility can prevent needless suffering. They also give one a feeling of well-being.

The exercises I describe in this book are highly efficient and take only a very short time to carry out. The total therapeutic program for the neck, described above, plus the jaw exercises that follow, take about three minutes and are in no way painful. If you do not suffer any limitation of movement in your neck or jaw,

I suggest that you do one five-minute session of these exercises once a week; do them regularly every Monday night. If, however, you do want to increase your range, add the five-minute exercise to the daily morning tense-relax-and-stretch program. You may add one other session of five minutes in the middle of the day, whenever convenient.

THE JAW

Exercises for the jaw joint, figures 29–32

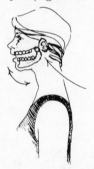

29. The jaw joint (Temporomandibular joint)

□ The joint which connects the jaw to the cranium, the temporomandibular joint, is located near the ear (fig. 29). You can pinpoint the exact location by moving your jaw up and down and pressing a fingertip firmly into your cheek. Anyone who has rheumatoid arthritis will not need to search long if there has been an involvement in that joint (involvement meaning inflammation, pain, redness, swelling, and heat). I have had many such involvements on both sides of the face, not necessarily at the same time. I noticed that they occurred sometimes after I had opened my mouth very wide to bite off a piece of food—as in eating an apple or a thick sandwich. Sometimes the involvement followed a visit to my dentist, where I had to open my mouth wide for treatment. The pain during such involvements was very severe, and seemed sometimes to come actually from the ear. I was able to control the pain and swelling by applying a small hot compress, then rubbing Ben-Gay or a similar ointment into the skin. No one ever suggested my doing exercises for this joint, which undoubtedly could have prevented much of the pain, since the involvement usually occurred after its sudden stretching. My experience is that if the joint range is maintained through exercise, an occasional opening of the mouth to the full range is less likely to result in pain and inflammation. As a matter of fact, since I started doing the jaw exercises, I have very rarely had an involvement of this joint.

My need to develop exercises for this joint occurred some twelve years after the onset of arthritis, when I developed a poor bite. I could not open my mouth wide enough to accept even a normal sandwich. The teeth also did not close in the front, so I could not bite off thin pieces of food, a condition called "open bite." Upper and lower molars no longer came together properly, which caused toothaches; I had to have a number of inlays replaced and teeth and fillings repeatedly ground down by the dentist so that the bite would remain in contact without undue pressure. This condition was looked at gravely by both my dentist and my rheumatologist. I started to consider the possibility of getting some benefit from exercises, but I could not find appropriate exercises described anywhere. I therefore adapted the same tense-relax-and-stretch system described above for the neck to the temporomandibular joints.

TESTING THE JAW RANGE

• Stand or sit in front of a mirror and open your mouth as wide as possible (fig. 30). Does it look as if you are opening your mouth wide enough? There is no definite rule as to how wide you should be able to open your mouth, but I would say that you should be able to open it at least 1 inch (2.5 cm), so that you can bite into a thick sandwich or a large apple.

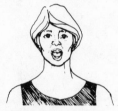

30. *Open mouth as wide as possible.*

EXERCISING THE JAW RANGE

• The exercise itself consists of contracting your chewing muscles by biting into a rod-shaped piece of wood, such as a kitchen spoon handle about ⅜ inch in diameter (8 mm) (fig. 31). Hold the pressure for two to three seconds (count of six), then release for a second or two and observe whether you are able to open your mouth a little wider (fig. 32). If you gain range, repeat the exercise at least once more.

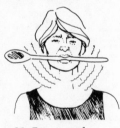

31. *Bite into the wooden spoon handle to the count of six, relax.*

After you have done the exercise a few times, you should learn to contract your chewing muscles without actually biting into anything. Just pretend you are biting by tensing the jaw muscles. A yawning motion has a similar exercising effect, since when you yawn the muscles contract to hold the joint in place.

This exercise actually increased the opening of my mouth, to the delight of my dentist. The problem of proper molar contact disappeared, as well as the pain from the involvements. I have since learned about the facial pain clinic directed by Dr. Joseph Marbach at the Columbia University School of Dentistry in New

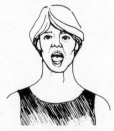

32. *Attempt to open your mouth a bit further.*

York City. In an article on facial pain and the temporomandibular joint (see Bibliography, section 7), Dr.
Marbach wrote that exercises are the best way to eliminate facial pain and discomfort. I found this to be true
in my own case.

Exercises for the arthritic jaw are rarely described
in the literature on the subject. In the Yoga system,
there is an exercise called "the Lion." You open your
mouth wide and stick your tongue out all the way.
Biomechanically speaking, by opening the mouth you
train and relax the muscles necessary for performing
that motion.

I came across a similar exercise in an airline in-flight
booklet. The command here is to open the mouth wide
and "shout" without actually uttering a sound. This,
again, is an isometric exercise for opening the temporomandibular joint. Both these exercises are good for
muscle relaxation and for stretching the mouth opening. For normal people, they are prophylactic (preventive) rather than therapeutic.

TENSE-RELAX-AND-STRETCH

☐ If you have been able to carry out the above exercises as described, you will have gained some insight
into the mechanics of isometric exercise, in which
there is muscle contraction without movement of the
joint, with the result that heat is produced inside the
muscle. This warm-up relaxes the muscles and allows
them to be extended more easily to their fullest possible range. For the arthritic, isometric contraction as
a relaxation procedure is highly preferable to any
strenuous repetitive motion. Subjecting arthritic joints
to wear and tear should be avoided; we want to con-
serve our joints as well as our energy. We use them
sparingly for those efforts that are really needed.

After you have carried out the neck exercises a number of times in the course of a week, you will probably
be able to do the isometric muscle contraction without
the opposing-hand resistance. We all know that we
can tense our upper arm muscle (biceps) to show off
our strength; this is often called "muscle setting" in
muscle exercise therapy. After we have learned to
tense our neck muscles by contracting them individually in various directions of motion of the head
against the opposing hand, we may omit the resisting

hands altogether. To stop the bending of the neck or rotating of the head at a certain point, we just stiffen our neck with a very slight motion to resist the imaginary hands. It helps to watch yourself in a mirror as you do this.

I hope you will practice this faithfully, since it can serve you as an efficient and time-saving technique in exercises to relax and stretch all the other parts of the body.

The tense-relax-and-stretch technique can produce strengthening if performed daily. I have not mentioned this aspect because weakness of the neck muscles does not seem to be a problem; I have found that the *tense-relax-and-stretch* exercises described above have helped me to keep my neck sufficiently strong. However, isometric strengthening applied to the finger, arm, or leg muscles can be of great importance, as we will see in subsequent chapters.

Note: For information about how you can obtain the devices and special equipment mentioned in this chapter, consult the Directory of Aids.

7 Tuesday Night: Shoulders and Elbows

☐ The shoulder is the most mobile joint of the human body. Its wide range of motion is accomplished through joints that connect the shoulder blade (scapula), upper arm (humerus), collar bone (clavicle), with the rib cage and sternum. To ensure that the many muscles involved in shoulder motion will glide smoothly over one another, small liquid-filled sacs called bursas are interposed between them. These bursas act like roller bearings; they reduce friction and facilitate smooth motion.

TESTING THE SHOULDER AND ELBOW RANGES

Testing the ranges of the shoulders and elbows, figures 1–13

☐ Possibly your range of shoulder motion has been limited to some degree, especially if there have been joint flare-ups. It is important to maintain the range of motion necessary for functioning in daily life. Try the following movements to see how close you can come to the full range of motion for this joint.

Testing the Ranges of Motion

• One range of motion of the shoulder is shown in fig. 1. Sit or stand in front of a mirror. If you have difficulty raising your arms by yourself, ask someone to

1. Raise arms forward and way up beyond the head. Then swing arms down and backward as far as possible.

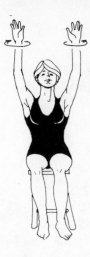

2. *Rotate arms so that palms face forward.*

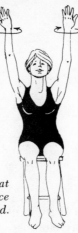

3. *Rotate arms so that backs of hands face forward.*

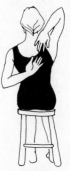

4. *Reach over the shoulder and behind the back, attempting to touch the fingertips.*

help you. Stop movements before they become painful. The arms are raised forward and up, over the head, then moved down and back, behind the body. When you reach the highest point with the arms, rotate them so that first palms and then backs of hands are facing the mirror (figs. 2, 3).

• In figure 4 the limits are tested as you attempt to reach all parts of your back. Reach over the shoulder with one hand and up from the waist, behind the back, with the other.

Complementary Movement: Reverse positions of the arms (fig. 5).

• Sitting or standing in front of a mirror, raise your arms straight out at sides with palms down (fig. 6). Then rotate palms up and raise your arms until they touch your ears. If you cannot quite succeed in doing this, raise first one arm and then the other arm. Lower the arms to right angles with the body and rotate so that first palms and then backs of hands face upward (fig. 7). Relax, bring arms down to your side.

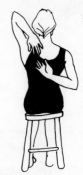

5. *Now reach with opposite hands.*

7. *Rotate arms to turn palms downward, then upward.*

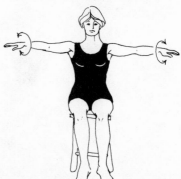

6. *Raise both arms sideways. Continue up until arms touch ears. Try one arm at a time, if you cannot do it with both together. As you raise arms past shoulder level, turn palms in.*

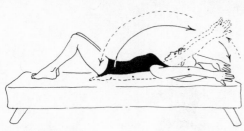

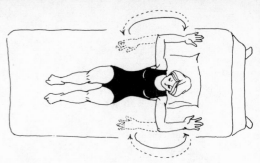

8. *Move arms up above head, and lower until thumbs touch the surface of the bed. Keep elbows straight.*

9. *Rotate upper arms by swinging hands up and down against the bed.*

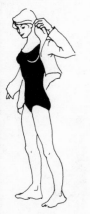

10. *When putting on a coat, you raise your arm sideways and rotate your shoulders forward.*

• If it is difficult for you to raise your arms without assistance, try raising your arms over your head while lying on the bed (fig. 8). Keep elbows as straight as possible. A variation, with elbows bent, is shown in fig. 9. This will rotate the arms. In daily activities (for example, getting into a coat) you need to raise the arms sideways and to rotate both arms. Some activities require reaching to your back, and frequently the elbows have to be bent (fig. 10). Slipping an undershirt over your head, or closing a zipper at the back of the neck, involves elbow flexion and elevation of the arm to reach behind the head.

• When you moved your arms all the way up at the side, you may have noticed that your arms had some difficulty in moving straight up; they tended to move somewhat forward, especially when you were about three-quarters through the range. In order to test this range properly, assume the position shown in figure 11. Place the palms of your hands against the back of your head, and move the elbows as far back as possible. They should reach beyond the shoulders.

• To test the ability to flex the elbows properly, place the palms of your hands behind your neck. Move elbows together until they touch (fig. 12). Avoid pain in any of the above positions; move only as far as you can with comfort. The positions shown illustrate the normal range that you want to achieve.

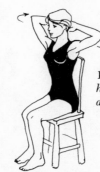

11. *Place hands behind head and elbows back as far as possible.*

12. *Place hands behind the neck, swing arms forward so that elbows touch.*

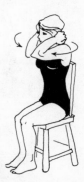

• Figure 13 shows movement of the straight arm in a wide circle. This circling motion is called movement of circumduction.

Complementary Movement: Perform circle with other arm.

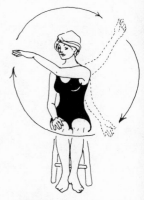

13. *Move the arm around in as large a circle as possible.*

If you can reach to the full range of motion in every direction, it is probably sufficient for you to exercise as described above. Move the arms several times in each direction. From the starting position move them all the way up, then rotate hands and swing down, as shown in figures 1–3. Next, raise your arms sideways to right angles to the body (fig. 7) and rotate hands. Bring arms down to the sides. Repeat these exercises a few times.

Each joint of the body should be exercised at least once a day to maintain range of motion. When I first started doing shoulder and arm exercises, I felt a lot of pain in my shoulders when I raised my arms. It was still important to go to the end of the range, however, and I found I could do this more easily for most exercises while lying down. In this position there is less gravitational pull to overcome as you move your arms sideways or beyond your head.

At one time, I found swimming an extremely efficient and pleasant way to maintain the range of motion of the shoulders and preserve strength in my arms, but I was not able to swim regularly. After about three years of arthritis, I had to discontinue cold water swimming. For those who can swim in the ocean or swimming pools on a regular basis, and for whom the cold water poses no risk, there is nothing better for keeping the shoulders and arms flexible and strong. And, of course, swimming in the warm waters of thermal pools, which is possible at many spas, is highly beneficial, provided the exercise is carried out on a daily basis.

PREPARATION FOR EXERCISE

☐ It is useful to warm up for the exercises with a bath or shower; they can even be performed while you are taking a hot shower, if you are stable enough on your feet. (When coming out of the bath or shower, be sure not to get chilled.)

Another way to warm up is to use a large electric heating pad across your back and shoulders for five minutes. I used the Thermophore moist hot pack. This pad is not controlled by a thermostat with low, medium, and high positions, but by a pushbutton that permits the pad to become as hot as you can stand.

Try to exercise in a room with at least 70°F (21°C) temperature. If you can take daily medication for pain or inflammation, take it half an hour before you do the exercises. I do not, however, advise exercising beyond the point of pain, although a slight amount of pain may be permissible in passive stretching of the limbs under supervision of a therapist. Also, when I do stretching with the aid of an overhead gym bar, I permit myself a small amount of pain; if I experience momentary pain from straining against the bar, I release the bar and thereby avoid causing persistent pain.

THE POSSIBLE MOTIONS

In order to understand the movement taking place at any joint of the extremities (arms and legs), let us observe that they can be bent or held straight (flexed or extended), moved away from or toward the center line of the body (abducted or adducted), and rotated outward or inward (externally or internally rotated).

I have already mentioned before how to test your range of motion in every direction (figs. 1–13). The purpose of the following exercises is to help you reach the fullest range of motion possible without experiencing pain.

TENSE-RELAX-AND-STRETCH EXERCISES FOR THE SHOULDER

□ Most of the stretching exercises can be done while lying down on the bed. Some exercises, however, are best done while you are either sitting or standing.

• Lie on the bed, using only a small pillow under the head, or no pillow at all if it is comfortable. Raise arms straight up in the air and then reach with arms straight back beyond your head to touch the bed with thumbs pointing down (fig. 8). The weight of the arm helps somewhat to bring it to the limit of the possible range. If you cannot reach the desired limit properly, work with one arm at a time. You may relax the muscles first before again attempting to reach the end of the range by slowly and repeatedly moving the arm through the full range—bringing it straight up, moving it past the ninety-degree angle, then bringing it back down to your side. This repeated movement is an isotonic exercise that warms up and relaxes the shoulder muscles.

- If the movement described in the preceding exercise causes you discomfort, warm up the muscles with isometric rather than isotonic exercises. The isometric exercise is performed near the end of the achievable range in the opposite direction. This means that you contract the antagonist muscles for two to three seconds (count of six), then relax briefly (one second), then attempt to move the arm a little farther in the desired direction to extend the range.

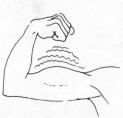

14. *Observe your biceps as you tense it.*

Tense-relax-and-stretch exercises for the shoulder, figures 15–21

15. *Push arm down against the hands of a helper for a count of six. Relax for one second, move arm upward, and repeat exercise.*

What I have just described is a muscle-tensing (also called muscle-setting) exercise without any motion of the joint. We have all seen how body builders flex the biceps to demonstrate strength (fig. 14). This is a typical muscle-tensing isometric exercise. However, without experience it is difficult for us to know exactly which muscle to flex for the purpose of extending the range of a particular shoulder movement. To gain this experience, it is good to work at first with a therapist or a helper who will help you to do this type of exercise against his or her resisting hand.

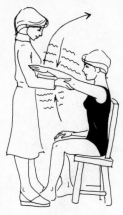

- Figure 15 shows how, in straight, forward arm-raising, the arm is pushed down as hard as possible against the hand of the therapist for a count of six, then relaxed for one second, then moved farther up. Figure 16 shows how the arm is moved up sideways as far as possible, then pressed against the resisting

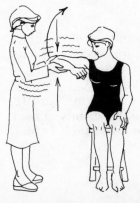

16. *Push arm down against the hands of a helper for a count of six. Relax for one second, move arm upward, and repeat exercise.*

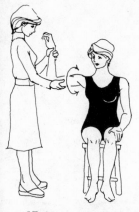

17. *Attempt to rotate the upper arm against the resistance of a helper for a count of six. Relax for a second, then attempt to rotate the arm in both directions as far as possible. Repeat exercises, figures 15–17 with other arm. Try to tense-relax-and-stretch without resistance by helper.*

hand of the therapist for a count of six, then relaxed and moved a little higher. Internal and external rotation of the arms can also be resisted, at the limit of rotation, by the two hands of the therapist (fig. 17) for a count of six, then relaxed for one second, then—if possible—rotated a little farther.

It is important to become aware which muscles are contracted when you are straining against the hands of the therapist or helper, or when doing the muscle-tensing exercises on your own (tensing your muscles as if you were moving your arm against a strong resistance in the direction opposite to the desired direction of improved range). The process may seem a little complicated at first, but you should be able to do it without difficulty after you have tried it a few times, especially if learned under the supervision of a therapist. I obtained my biggest reward from observing how I could extend the range of my shoulder joint or any other joint of the body through this method, which I call the *tense-relax-and-stretch* technique. The same form of exercise, carried out against resistance, is well known to therapists as the hold-relax technique of the PNF (proprioceptive neuromuscular facilitation) system. I have adapted it for home use by arthritics by replacing the isometric exercise against external resistance with a muscle-tensing (setting) exercise. Of course, it is best to learn this technique with a therapist, but if you are working alone, remember that frequent repetition and complete understanding are necessary before it can become second nature. In this book, I frequently repeat biomechanical explanations so that you will understand how the isometric tensing of the muscles, followed by relaxation and then by stretching produces a wider joint range. Thus, you will know what is expected of you when you move to the next joint and repeat the procedure.

Complementary Exercise

• Repeat the isometric tense-relax-and-stretch exercise with the other arm, moving the arm up or sideways above the head, and also rotating it (figs. 15–17).

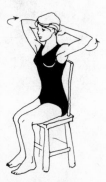

18. *Place hands behind head and elbows back as far as possible.*

• In order to increase the range indicated in figure 18, sit on the chair with the palms of the hands in back of your head. Your helper or therapist stands behind

Tuesday Night: Shoulders and Elbows

the chair and moves the elbows gently back. Indicate when you reach the point of slightest discomfort. At this point, press strongly forward against the resisting hand as hard as possible to a count of six. You will notice that muscles across your chest, the pectorals, are strained. You relax for a second, after which the helping hands move your elbows slowly back to extend the range.

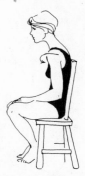

19. *Tense shoulders as if to move muscles forward.*

I usually experienced a considerable expansion of range, especially when I hadn't done this exercise for a while. Few motions in daily life stretch the pectorals other than the deliberate stretching described here, and so they tend to become tight. You should repeat this exercise a number of times with your helper until you feel that you have reached the possible limit of range. After you have become aware of the muscle groups that need strengthening, try to tighten them by muscle tensing without the resistance of a helper, then relax for one second and stretch your arms out in the desired direction as far as you can. You may notice that at first you do not achieve as much range as when working with a helper. This is because you may not be contracting the pectoral muscles as strongly without resistance as with resistance (it took me a number of trials until I felt I was contracting the muscles as powerfully when tensing them as when straining against resistance). Another reason is that the agonist muscles, which produce motion in the desired direction, may not be strong enough to overcome the tightness of the antagonist muscles—in this case, the pectorals; they will have to be trained by isometric or isotonic exercises (which are described below).

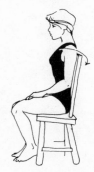

20. *Relax, roll shoulders back.*

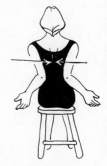

21. *Pull shoulder blades together to the count of six.*

• To do the range-of-motion exercise without a helper (figures 18–20), tense your chest muscles, as if to bring elbows together, for the count of six, relax, then press the shoulder blades together, bringing elbows out and back as far as possible for a count of six (fig. 21).

PASSIVE STRETCHING TO EXTEND RANGES

□ When we do the isometric tense-relax-and-stretch exercises, we arrive at a certain limit, but not at the *final* limit of range. There may be some tissues around the joint that can be passively stretched, or slight tissue adhesions which can be broken. When I carry out muscle stretching to the limit daily, I find that the range slowly increases. This increase in range can be speeded up by gentle manipulation or by passive stretching. This is best done by a therapist who will exercise judgment about how far you can go in your range without developing persistent pain. In passive stretching you must expect to feel some pain at the limit of range; this should pass when the stretching is stopped, but persistent pain means that you have to rest the joint in order to recover. Judging how far you can move a joint without developing persistent pain is something of an art in which therapist and patient co-operate. Patients' responses to pain differ, so the decision is not easy.

When *therapists* move a joint passively through its range, they refer to this procedure as *stretching;* it produces results in the relatively brief time that patient and therapist are able to work together. I like to call this procedure *manipulative stretching,* or *manipulation.* For the active stretching that I describe in this book, at the end of each isometric tense-relax-and-stretch exercise, I prefer the simple term *stretching* used in its everyday sense; this is the type of exercise most suitable for a patient in a home program. There are a few positions in which manipulative stretching can be carried out by the patient without the aid of a therapist. This can be productive, but we have to be careful and develop skill in judging for ourselves how far to go short of causing persistent pain. I will describe this later with the use of the gym bar (chinning bar).

EXERCISES FOR ELBOW FLEXION

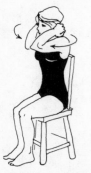

• This exercise for complete elbow flexion is convenient to do following the one described in figure 11 above, in which the elbows were bent back.

Slide both hands down from the back of your head to the back of your neck (fig. 22). Swing elbows slowly forward until elbows touch. If you have difficulty reaching the full range (elbows touching), repeat slowly, stop at the end of the range, hold elbows very stiff for a count of six, relax and try to move farther.

22. *Place hands behind the neck, swing arms forward so that elbows touch.*

Tuesday Night: Shoulders and Elbows

- There is one other way to exercise elbow flexion, which I used as long as my wrists were flexible. Flex your elbows and raise your hands to touch both shoulders (fig. 23); this tests flexibility both of the elbow and of the wrists. If the wrists do not flex properly, you will be unable to reach your shoulders, even though elbows flex properly. After you have touched your shoulders with your elbows hanging down, try to move your elbows up so that the forearms are in a horizontal position while your hands or fingertips are still touching your shoulders (fig. 24).

- Next, an exercise to stretch the elbows. You will have observed, while stretching your arms straight up, whether the elbows are straight. If they are not, do the following tense-relax-and-stretch exercise with them, first with the aid of a therapist or helper. The helper's hand grasps your lower arm, and tries to straighten the elbow. When you come to the end of the range, bend the elbow as strongly as possible against the resisting hand of the helper, to the count of six. Relax for a second. The helper now moves the forearm to extend the elbow further. Repeat this procedure a few times, as long as you feel there is a slight gain in range of motion. Repeat the same exercise with the other arm.

   The muscle that contracts during the isometric part of the exercise is the biceps. Whenever you want to straighten your elbow, remember that you can facilitate this by first flexing the biceps.

- You can also exercise passively to straighten the elbow. While sitting on a chair, bend forward and place the lower left arm between the legs in such a way that the left wrist pushes against your right leg just below the knee, and the arm just below the elbow presses against the left thigh (fig. 25a). Now, contract the biceps by pressing the wrist strongly against your right leg for a count of six. Relax for one second. Now move both knees slowly together to straighten the elbow, as in fig. 25b. *Be careful!* This is a passive exercise; it is very tempting to try to straighten out your elbow by force. If you are too enthusiastic and impatient about it, you could develop persistent pain. Stop when you have straightened the elbow to the point of pain. It is better to repeat the exercise a few times than to go about it too vigorously.

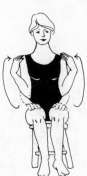

23. *Bring arms up and touch shoulders with fingertips.*

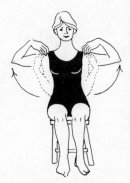

24. *Now try to move elbows up, so arms are horizontal.*

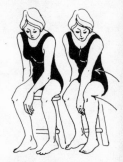

25a. *Place lower arm between thighs and knees. Tense biceps, and relax.*

25b. *Draw knees together to straighten the elbow.*

Complementary Exercise

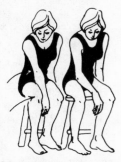

26a & 26b. *Repeat with the other arm if needed.*

• Straighten your right elbow by placing your right forearm between your legs (fig. 26a) so that your right wrist touches the left leg just below the knee and the arm just below the elbow is pressed against the right thigh. Contract the biceps by pressing the wrist strongly against the left leg for a count of six. Relax for one second. Now move legs slowly together to straighten the elbow until you come to the limit of range (fig. 26b). Repeat a few times moving legs closer together to further straighten the elbow, as long as you can gain a little more range each time without undue pain.

THE CHINNING BAR FOR SHOULDER AND ELBOW STRETCHING

☐ Both elbows and shoulders can be stretched by using the chinning bar. I have used one, installed between a door frame, satisfactorily for many years. You can make your own, of course, but a bar of the telescoping type, which can be easily repositioned as you make progress in reaching higher, is well worth the investment (see Directory of Aids).

• Install the chinning bar where you can just barely reach it with your fingertips while your feet are flat on the floor (fig. 27). Now raise yourself onto your toes and grasp the bar over the top (fig. 28). While holding tightly to the bar, slowly lower your heels to

Stretching shoulders and elbows, figures 27–41

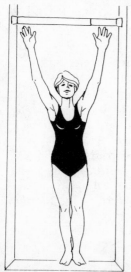

27. *Install a chinning bar so that you can barely touch it, standing with feet flat on floor.*

28. *Rise onto the toes, grasp bar, slowly lower the heels to the floor.*

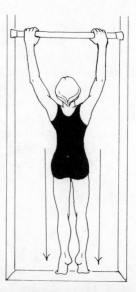

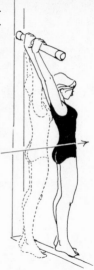

the floor. This produces a passive stretch in the elbows and shoulders. Be careful not to stretch too suddenly! Lower your heels very slowly. If at any point you experience pain which you feel might persist, release your hold on the bar. Gentle repetition of this exercise will help extend your elbow and shoulder ranges.

- You can also stretch arms and shoulders backward with the following tense-relax-and-stretch exercise (fig. 29). Strain forward against the bar with your hands for a count of six, relax for one second, then slowly walk forward a few inches at a time while still holding onto the bar. Avoid pain in doing this.

REGAINING STRENGTH AFTER BED REST

□ My shoulder range has decreased noticeably during periods of enforced bed rest. On getting back to work with the chinning bar, I had to lower it, but usually I could regain the original height in a week or two of daily stretching, limiting stretches to a few seconds' duration. Whenever I passed through the doorway where the bar was, I grasped the bar for a few seconds and then let go.

After a period of enforced bed rest quite independent of arthritis, I found that my shoulder strength had decreased considerably. The deltoid muscle, a triangular-shaped muscle covering the top of the shoulder that acts in lifting the arm in all directions (fig. 30),

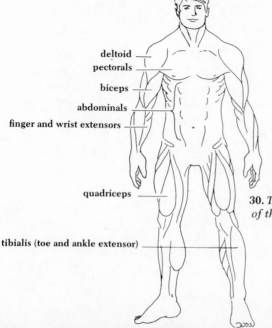

deltoid
pectorals
biceps
abdominals
finger and wrist extensors

quadriceps

tibialis (toe and ankle extensor)

30. *The triangular deltoid muscle, covering the top of the shoulder, and active in lifting the arm in all various directions, can become quite weak.*

had evidently become quite weak. Inability to reach a chinning bar after a period of inactivity may be due primarily to weakness rather than loss of joint range.

PASSIVE EXERCISES FOR PAINFUL SHOULDERS

☐ According to *The Arthritis Reporter* (New York Chapter, no. 1, 1977), the vulnerability of the shoulder stems from the time man decided to walk on two legs instead of four and began to raise his arms during daily activities. In our present state of evolution, the design of the shoulder joint is not yet fully suited to such use. The supraspinatus tendon can become damaged, and both the sheath surrounding it and the lubricating sac, or bursa, nearby can become inflamed (bursitis). The inflammation musters a large army of white blood cells to repair the damage. In the body's overzealous effort at self-repair, adhesions—actually scar tissue—may develop between various tissues and limit the range of motion of the shoulder. If left untreated, the condition can result in what is aptly described as a "frozen shoulder." To prevent such adhesions, gentle exercises to put the shoulder passively through all of its ranges should be performed at least once daily. Active exercises are not possible in this stage, since in any motion to raise the arm the supraspinatus tendon has to exercise a pull, and in its inflamed condition, this will cause acute pain. I have had several short-lived episodes of this sort, in which passive exercises of the type described in figures 31 and 32 below were quite successful.

• Here is the pendulum exercise for passive shoulder movement (fig. 31). Bend your body forward, leaning with your "good" arm on a table. With the other arm describe pendulum motions—forward, backward, sideways, and *in a circle*—within the limits of pain.

After the pain due to the bursitis or tendonitis has subsided, active exercise may be resumed.

There is also a system of passive exercises for the shoulder that uses a pulley. I will describe it although I was never very successful with it; I experienced immoderate pain, probably due to the severe inflam-

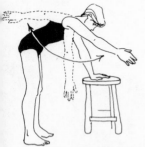

31. *Pendulum swing arm forward, backward, and sideways, as well as in a circle. Repeat with other arm if necessary.*

Tuesday Night: Shoulders and Elbows

matory condition of my shoulders. However, the following exercise may be useful for people who do not have such a severe and prolonged shoulder involvement as I had.

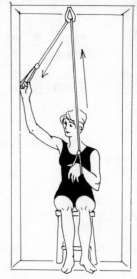

- The apparatus for the pulley consists of a single pulley attached to a bracket at the top of the doorframe. A piece of clothesline is fed through the pulley (or around the hook) and the ends of the line are looped to facilitate holding it in the hands. The length of the line is adjusted so that when you sit on a chair below the pulley and pull all the way down with one hand, the other hand will be pulled all the way up (fig. 32).

  This exercise system can be effective when only one shoulder is involved and painful. The healthy arm and hand can keep pulling the affected arm up and down; and the affected arm can also lean in various directions and be pulled. In this way, various limits of range can be approached. If both arms are affected, my experience is that such an exercise soon becomes very uncomfortable.

32. *Using a pulley, the healthy arm can exercise the passive, affected arm.*

Instead of a pulley or hook, one can also hang the line over the top of the gym bar. Pulley exercise sets are available at surgical supply stores. An advantage of these is that comfortable handles are supplied. In rehabilitation gyms you may encounter pulleys with adjustable weights attached. Such a system can be useful if adapted, in a simplified form, to your home program. But remember this limitation about weighted pulleys: Although working with them gives you the sense of strengthening your arms, you are not strengthening those muscles that raise your arms, which is mostly what is needed.

I sometimes have difficulty raising an arm up to the gym bar (I then give it an assist with my other hand). Building strength for this can be done by "walking" your fingers up the doorframe, using friction between the fingertips and the frame to prevent the arm from falling down (fig. 33). If need be, you can help your arm with the other hand. I have seen, in a rehabilitation institute, a type of finger ladder that can be used for this purpose (fig. 34). The arm moves up very slowly as the fingers climb the ladder. Weak muscles are helped by the support of the fingers on the steps of the ladder.

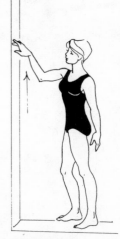

33. *Walk fingers up a door frame to strengthen weak muscles.*

34. *Walk up a finger ladder.*

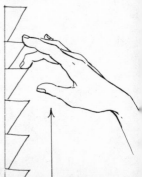

SHOULDER EXERCISES FOR BETTER POSTURE

☐ The following exercises will loosen those muscles that make your shoulders feel tight and prevent you from assuming a good posture. Do these exercises in front of a mirror for the first time, so that you can check whether you are doing them correctly. Once you observe them, learn them, and know what they are for, you will not need the mirror anymore.

• With arms at your sides, raise shoulders slowly, steadily, as if you were straining against resistance, as high as possible (fig. 35). Avoid moving your head downward while performing this exercise.

Next, let your shoulders drop all the way down while pulling the head straight up, with chin in and neck back (fig. 36).

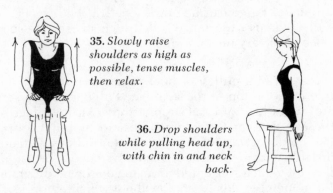

35. *Slowly raise shoulders as high as possible, tense muscles, then relax.*

36. *Drop shoulders while pulling head up, with chin in and neck back.*

Now produce round shoulders by moving them forward and in (fig. 37). Again this motion is slow and deliberate, as if you were straining against resistance.

Now, rotate shoulders backward and pinch shoulder blades together as hard as you can. Remain in this position to at least the count of six (fig. 38). (This

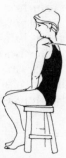

37. *Round the shoulders by moving them forward and in.*

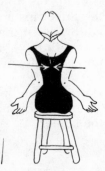

38. *Pull shoulder blades together to the count of six.*

position is conducive to good posture, and an isometric tense-relax-and-stretch exercise for it is described in chapter 9.)

Now rotate the shoulders through a full circle, first in the forward direction (fig. 39), and then in a backward direction. Do this several times.

We need not only range of motion but also strength to carry out daily activities. If we have been pulling our sweaters off, drying our backs with towels (fig. 40), and putting our coats on by ourselves all our lives (fig. 41), we are surprised to find that we can no longer do such things with ease once arthritis has struck. Our instinct seems to tell us to exercise these motions repeatedly and thereby maintain function. Thus, when you start having difficulty putting your coat on, you are likely to redouble your efforts rather than ask someone to help you. But we all know this doesn't work. The answer lies in deliberate strengthening exercises.

Ideally, strengthening should be done for each muscle separately, using isometric exercises for highest efficiency in various parts of the range. However, the shoulder is such a complicated joint, involving so many bones and so many crisscrossing muscles (fig. 42), that a program of exercises for all the different muscles in the different parts of their range is simply not practical. Nevertheless, I believe that some degree of biomechanical understanding is required, not only to help you comprehend the various isometric exer-

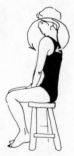

39. Shoulders shrugging and circling forward and backward.

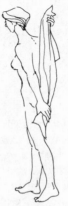

40. Strength and range of motion can be exercised in daily activities, such as drying your back with a towel.

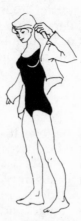

41. Elbow flexion with raised arm when putting on coat.

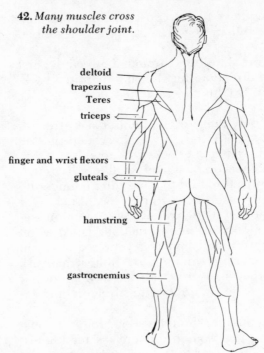

42. *Many muscles cross the shoulder joint.*

deltoid
trapezius
Teres
triceps

finger and wrist flexors
gluteals

hamstring

gastrocnemius

cise positions described here but, more importantly, to help you design your own isometric exercise positions for the shoulders and arms wherever you may be in the course of the day. Fortunately, the great mobility of the shoulder joint permits this. Whether you are lying down, sitting, or standing, you will always be able to reach with your arm, and press against the bed, a pillow, or a piece of furniture. If you do this for a count of six, you will have strengthened some muscles isometrically. But you want to activate all the muscles, so keep in mind that arms can be pushed up or down, left or right, rotated inward or outward—and all this at various positions in the range of motion.

YOUR PERSONALIZED EXERCISE PROGRAM

☐ I believe it is best to design an exercise regimen with the advice of a therapist, if you have one. If none is available, go through all exercises mentioned several times until you decide which of the stretching and isometric exercises are most useful to help you maintain range and strengthen muscles. Isometric exercises ought not to result in pain or exhaustion unless you repeat them too often or exercise too long. Also, isometric exercises can be carried out—and are even recommended—during the acute phase of rheumatoid arthritis, when much rest is indicated. Confirm this, however, with your doctor.

I recommend a definite five- to ten-minute program of shoulder exercise to be done once weekly, let us say, Tuesday night. Allotting a definite time is the best insurance that the exercises will be done. If arms and shoulders require more than usual attention because of weakness, this program can also be done following your daily five-minute morning tense-relax-and-stretch exercises. And it can be done a second time during the course of the day. On whatever night you choose, do all of the range-of-motion exercises and as many isometric exercises as you can fit in within ten minutes. After a while, you will become accustomed to the isometric exercises and will intersperse them with the individual range-of-motion exercises. What is more, you will become aware that each range-of-motion exercise "contains" an isometric exercise for the antagonist muscle—the muscle pulling in the opposite direction from the intended direction of motion. You may also then add an isometric exercise for the agonist muscle—the muscle pulling in the intended direction of motion. Finally, you will have learned so much about your arm and shoulder musculature that you will be able to voluntarily contract various muscles of your shoulders and arms (fig. 42), somewhat in the way that body builders flex their muscles. This type of exercise can be done conveniently at any time and place during the day, whether you are in the shower, sitting in an airplane, or standing on line.

MORE ISOMETRICS FOR STRENGTHENING

☐ Aside from the exercises described earlier, there are helpful isometric exercises you can do using a ball or a belt. In others you use your own arm or leg to provide resistance. Finally, I describe a group to do using furniture.

In all these exercises remember that the following pattern is repeated:

1. Arms up
2. Arms down

3. Arms sideways
4. Arms turned inward
5. Arms turned outward

In the first group of exercises that follow I have chosen an *inflatable beach ball* and a *latex rubber belt* because both have a certain amount of "give (a leather belt may be used, but it permits only pure isometric exercise, with no movement of the joints)." You might at first suppose that the resulting exercises will be isotonic rather than isometric because of the movement involved in compressing the rubber ball or expanding the rubber belt. However, maximum energy is expended only at the end of the movement of compression or expansion. At that point, joints do not move anymore, and the isometric contraction takes place. Before reaching that point, in the process of compressing or expanding, relatively little strength is expended, but the movement stimulates nerve endings around the joint, sending signals along neuromuscular pathways and thereby reinforcing the strength of contraction and making the exercise more efficient. If the rubber belt is not tight enough, you may not reach a point of very strong resistance, and will thereby carry out an isotonic exercise. Though not as efficient as the isometric one, it will produce some strengthening.

Data obtained in clinical studies of isometric strengthening exercises for fingers show that patients directed to exercise "as strongly as possible" without any further explanation will apply approximately twice the strength they would normally use in performing the action. If this ratio applies as well to muscles moving the upper extremities, it would mean, for example, that if we are accustomed to lifting weights of five pounds with a certain extension of the arm, we will, at the command to exercise as strongly as possible, lift against the resistance of the rubber belt with the equivalent of a weight of ten pounds. Exercising this way repeatedly twice a day for three seconds (count of six) will probably give the greatest possible daily gain in strength. Exercising once a week will help to maintain strength.

If we have particularly painful joints, it may not be possible to exercise at twice the strength used in daily activities; merely carrying out the activities themselves may be difficult. In this case, we can still accomplish strengthening through many repetitions of the exercise, let us say, ten or twenty times for three seconds (count of six) at normal strength.

We can effectively strengthen the muscles of the upper extremities by exercising them as hard as possible isometrically, twice a day for three seconds (count of six), or once a day for six seconds (count of twelve). We can maintain strength by exercising once weekly.

I use a thirty-eight-inch (one meter) circumference beach ball. If you want to use the same beach ball for exercising the leg muscles, be sure it is a size that fits comfortably between your knees. The rubber belt can be obtained from a surgical supply store (see Glossary of Aids), or it can be fashioned from six-inch-wide (fifteen centimeters) "dental dam," available from dental supply companies. One square yard of six-inch (15 cm) dental dam furnishes two pieces forty-four inches (1.13 meters) long; knot the ends of one piece to make a belt. If stronger resistance is desired, place the two pieces on top of each other and then knot the ends.

Exercising with a Beach Ball

• With the ball at shoulder level and out to one side squeeze it for three seconds (count of six, fig. 43). Switch to the other side and repeat. Hold the ball in front of you with one arm on top and the other arm below (fig. 44); squeeze for three seconds (count of six).

Now rotate the ball back so the other arm is on top

Isometric strengthening exercises, figures 43–61

43. *Hold a beach ball to each side squeezing as hard as possible for three seconds.*

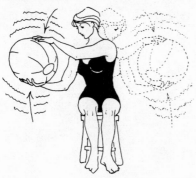

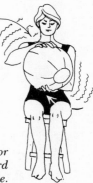

44. *Squeeze ball for three seconds as hard as possible.*

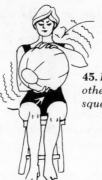

45. *Rotate ball so that other arm is on top and squeeze.*

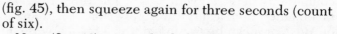

46. *Squeeze ball tightly against abdomen for a count of six.*

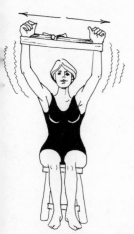

47. *Holding arms as high as possible, strain outward against a looped latex rubber belt for three seconds.*

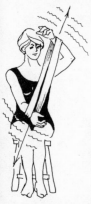

48. *Holding one arm as high as possible and the other below, strain strongly against the belt for three seconds.*

(fig. 45), then squeeze again for three seconds (count of six).

Next (fig. 46), press the ball against your body as strongly as possible for three seconds (count of six).

Exercising with a Rubber (or Leather) Belt

• Place the belt over forearms near the wrists, hold arms as high up as possible (fig. 47). Strain against the belt as strongly as possible for three seconds (count of six).

Now, hold one arm up high as possible and the other arm below (fig. 48). Strain as strongly as possible against the belt for three seconds (count of six).

Now, reverse arms so that the other arm is up (fig. 49). Strain as strongly as possible for three seconds (count of six).

Next, move arms down to waist level (fig. 50). Strain outward against the belt for three seconds (count of six).

• In the next series, you move *arms against arms, arms against legs.*

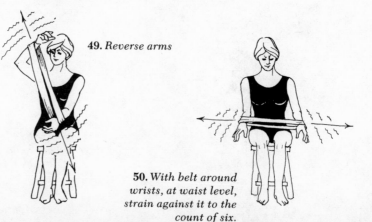

49. *Reverse arms*

50. *With belt around wrists, at waist level, strain against it to the count of six.*

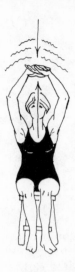

51. *Place right palm over back of left hand and press hands against one another strongly for three seconds.*

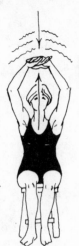

52. *Reverse position of hands and repeat exercise.*

Raise both arms up high, place right palm over the back of left hand (fig. 51). Press hands against each other as strongly as possible for three seconds (count of six).

Reverse hands so that left palm is over the back of the right hand (fig. 52). Press hands against each other as strongly as possible for three seconds (count of six).

Now, lower arms to shoulder level and place right palm over the back of the left hand (fig. 53). Press hands against each other as strongly as possible for three seconds (count of six).

Next, reverse hands so that the left palm is over the back of the right hand (fig. 54). Press hands against each other as strongly as possible for three seconds (count of six).

Place your arms so that the outer edges of your forearms are against the insides of your thighs just above the knees (fig. 55). Press your arms outward against the resisting thighs as strongly as possible for three seconds (count of six).

After relaxing for a few moments, place your arms around your thighs (fig. 56). Strain upward, as though attempting to lift your resisting legs, for three seconds (count of six).

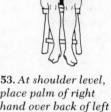

53. *At shoulder level, place palm of right hand over back of left hand and press hands against one another strongly for three seconds.*

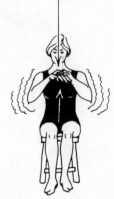

54. *Reverse hands and repeat exercise.*

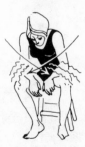

55. *Place forearms against thighs and press outward strongly for three seconds.*

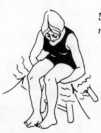

56. *Place arms around thighs and strain upward, as if attempting to lift legs, for three seconds.*

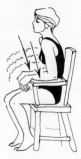

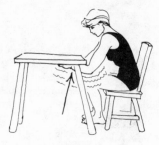

57. *Press forearms down on armrests for three seconds. Repeat with palms up.*

58. *Press with forearms against the underside of a table. Attempt with palms up and with palms down.*

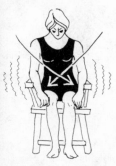

59. *Stem with forearms against the inner sides of armrests for a count of six.*

• Use your *chair or table to provide resistance* in the following exercises.

Sitting on a chair with armrests, press down with your forearms as strongly as possible for three seconds (count of six). Do this once with palms down (fig. 57) and once with palms up.

Press with your forearms against the underside of a table. Do this once with palms up and once with palms down (fig. 58), each time for a count of six.

Press with your forearms against the inner sides of the armrests. Do this each time for a count of six (fig. 59).

Keeping arms straight, press your hands as hard as you can down against the seat of your chair for a count of six (fig. 60).

While seated, grasp the underside of the chair seat and attempt to lift the chair, straining as strongly as possible, for a count of six (fig. 61).

After you have gained experience with the various groups of exercises, you can choose those exercises in each group that seem most suitable for your weekly (Tuesday evening?) exercise session. Once you have achieved sufficient body awareness and are able to feel the individual muscles contracting, you may substitute muscle-tensing exercises for the isometric exercises described. This saves time. You may also feel tempted at times during the day to tense your arm and shoulder muscles. This will be found to be very relax-

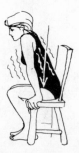

60. *Press, with arms straight down, as hard as possible against the seat of a chair.*

61. *Grasp underside of chair seat attempting to lift the chair. Strain as strongly as possible for a count of six.*

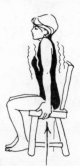

ing and at the same time it will help you maintain or
gain strength.

POSTSCRIPT 1: WEAKNESS AFTER BED REST

□ Several times during my years of arthritis, I have
had weakness in shoulder and arm muscles to such an
extent that isometric exercises did not seem efficient.
Usually this weakness was the aftermath of prolonged
bed rest. To regain strength, I did isotonic exercises
with weights.

The weights I used ranged from one pound to three
pounds. (One-pound weights are readily available in
the form of sugar or salt boxes. For the two- and three-
pound weights, I used the ankle weights I have for
strengthening the thigh muscles, available at surgical
supply stores.)

The isotonic lifting exercise consists of raising your
hand to shoulder level and then lifting it straight up
into the air. Repeat as many times as possible, up to
twenty times. Once you can lift both arms separately
twenty times as described, try to lift them while holding a one-pound weight in both hands, bringing the
weight up toward your head and then raising it
straight up over your head. Repeat this exercise until
you can do it twenty times (figs. 62a, 62b). Next lift the
one-pound weight with one arm as often as possible,
then do the same with the other arm.

After you can lift the one-pound weight twenty
times with each arm, repeat this procedure, first with
a two-pound ankle weight and then with a three-
pound ankle weight. Finally, put the weights into a
shopping bag and carry it for about fifteen feet, gradually increasing the weights to a load of ten pounds.

Do this exercise, like all the others, first with one
arm and then with the other arm, gradually progressing to heavier weights.

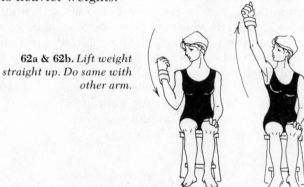

62a & 62b. *Lift weight
straight up. Do same with
other arm.*

After finishing this course of isotonic exercises (it took me a week; for others it may take more or less time), I continued the daily program of isometric exercises described earlier in the chapter. After about one to two months of daily isometric exercises, I continued with once-weekly isometric exercises.

POSTSCRIPT 2: PAINFUL ELBOWS

☐ When elbows were painful, I treated them for ten to twenty minutes with a hot soak or in a whirlpool bath (fig. 63), after which I either bandaged them loosely with Ace bandages, or slipped woollen elastic knee warmers over them. (When new, before they are stretched by the knees, these warmers can be used for the elbows.) It was particularly beneficial to leave the bandages or knee warmers on at night. In case of strong inflammation of the elbow, the Ace bandage is preferable, since it keeps the joint more immobile and therefore the joint is better rested.

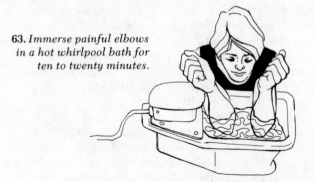

63. Immerse painful elbows in a hot whirlpool bath for ten to twenty minutes.

It never had occurred to me in the early years of arthritis, when I had frequent elbow involvements, that stability of the elbows someday would be very important in such actions as getting up or leaning on a cane. No particular finger strength is necessary for using a cane. Strength is transmitted through the elbow and shoulder, and these must be stable if the cane itself is to provide stability.

Note: For information about how you can obtain the devices and special equipment mentioned in this chapter, consult the Directory of Aids.

Wednesday Night: 8
Hands and Wrists

□ Every joint in the body serves an important purpose in its own way, yet the hands, with their complex interplay of joints, seem particularly important to us. We use our hands all the time, which means that if we don't have the use of our hands we are handicapped all the time.

In arthritis, the finger joints are attacked early, often before the disease is even diagnosed. In rheumatoid arthritis, the inflamed knuckles are vulnerable to destruction when fingers are used in their accustomed way; eventually the finger segments become twisted in odd directions and the fingers are unable to grasp. The muscles spanning the painful joints tend to waste, and as their supportive function lessens, deformities set in.

Medication is helpful to reduce inflammation and pain. However, a regimen of rest and exercises to strengthen the muscles can help delay the destruction of the knuckles by keeping the knuckles stabilized and minimizing abnormal pull. Fingers supported by strong muscles will not be immediately displaced when we lean against or carry an object with them.

The motions of the hands and wrists include flexion and extension, abduction and adduction, and internal and external rotation. Considering the large number

143

of finger joints, we might suppose that innumerable exercises would be needed to fully exercise them. This may well be the reason why comprehensive finger exercises were unavailable for so long. There were only a few standard exercises: making a fist; spreading the fingers apart; touching the tip of the thumb to the tips of the individual fingers; and placing the hand on a flat surface and lifting individual fingers. An exercise that arthritics should avoid is squeezing a rubber ball. It is destructive of the finger joints, and I personally find it inefficient, since pain in the knuckles prevents one from squeezing the rubber ball hard enough to produce a strengthening effect. The only other exercises for hands and fingers I know of are performing the so-called études for the piano (or just plain piano-playing) and the various hand and finger positions used by dancers and Yoga practitioners, which are intended mainly to achieve flexibility.

WHY AND HOW I DEVELOPED THE HAND GYM

□ My fingers became weak and clumsy one or two years before inflammation actually appeared. I lost the ability to use the precision tools that were necessary to my work. Even turning a key in a lock became more difficult, and opening a jar produced pain in the big knuckles. When inflammation of the knuckles began, I simply stopped using the painful fingers. As the inflammation subsided in these fingers and moved on to the other fingers, the whole hand gradually became very weak. During periods of remission for individual fingers, the muscles of these fingers never quite regained their strength since there was no way to train them individually, and the pain in the inflamed fingers made it very hard to do squeezing exercises for the whole hand. After about two years of the disease, my fingers seemed to stiffen at wrong angles, so that, besides lacking strength, they were now unable to grip things properly. I could no longer use a knife and fork, nor could I button my shirt and tie my shoelaces. My rheumatologist sent me to a hand surgeon who outlined to me the possibility of fusing some of the joints; the suggested procedure also would have "released" the overly strong contracture of some of the muscles to permit a better grip—though not necessarily more strength. (Nowadays finger joints can be replaced with

Silastic rubber implants, which produce a good-looking hand but only limited improvement in strength, if any.) I therefore studied the possibility of deliberate exercises to loosen some of my tight muscles. This seemed preferable to the so-called surgical release, by which some of the muscle mass or the associated tendinous structure would be removed and the muscles rendered less effective. I wanted to preserve the muscles as far as possible. I also realized that after an operation, strengthening would have to be done through deliberate exercise anyway. I therefore worked out my own exercise system, designing an apparatus which my wife, Elsa, put together, according to my instructions, out of cardboard, bolts, rubber bands, and foam rubber. I called it the Hand Gym. By placing my fingers in the straight slots, I counteracted their tendency to deviate in the direction of the little finger (ulnar deviation). I could press my fingers against the walls of the slots on both sides to increase strength (fig. 1). The bolts that passed through the walls at right angles provided support for the fingers to counteract the direction of deformity; that is, if the first segment beyond the large knuckle developed a tendency flexion, the bolt would support this segment in the extended position. Where the middle segment seemed to want to hyperextend or point upward (swan-neck deformity), I exercised the finger by trying to curl it around a foam-rubber roll.

Exercises of a few minutes' duration, several times a day, resulted in my regaining sufficient strength and flexibility to be able once again to feed and dress myself. I have maintained this ability now for twelve

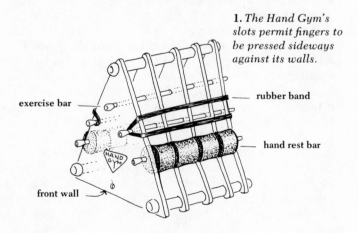

1. *The Hand Gym's slots permit fingers to be pressed sideways against its walls.*

exercise bar

rubber band

hand rest bar

front wall

years even though my hands are reduced in strength. Apparently, I was able to retard the process of deformation and retain sufficient strength, even if it is limited by the destruction the joints have suffered. We arthritics have to "live within the limitations" dictated by our joints. However, maintaining flexibility goes far in substituting for strength.

THE CLINICAL STUDIES

□ My rheumatologist, Dr. Otto Steinbrocker, was very pleased with the results I had obtained with the Hand Gym and asked me to explain the system to the doctors at the Institute of Rehabilitation Medicine at New York University Medical Center in New York City. The occupational therapy department and the clinical director of the institute, Dr. Edward Lowman, were quite excited about the possibilities of this exercise system. They undertook a two-year clinical study during which a booklet with detailed descriptions of the exercises was compiled by Doris Bens, an occupational therapist at the institute. The Hand Gym was then modified to fit the various sizes of hands, and one hundred were produced. At the institute it was also found that the exercises benefited people with weakness or partial paralysis from conditions other than arthritis, such as strokes, fractures, burns, and hand surgery. A manufacturer was found and today the Hand Gym is distributed through surgical and medical supply houses throughout the United States and in many other countries (catalogue number F70900, Maddak, Inc., Pequannock, N.J. 07440). The instructions are available in ten languages. The exercises in this chapter are designed to be done with the Hand Gym. If you are in treatment, ask your doctor or therapist to supervise your first exercise session. In a few instances, the principles behind certain exercises can be adapted for exercising without the Hand Gym. I am offering this system here because, as I have said, it is the only fully balanced regimen of hand exercises that I know of.

While the instructions were being compiled at the institute, I did some studies of the electrical impulses of finger muscles during their contraction to see in what directions isometric contractions (without joint motion) would be most efficient for strengthening. I also dissected hands together with Dr. Steinbrocker, at New York University Medical School, to get more insight into the function of finger muscles. I did extensive bibliographical research on finger deformities and exercises in arthritis and presented a summary of my design and analysis to Dr. Adrian Flatt, a renowned hand surgeon who specializes in arthritis cases. In his critique, he supported the concept and advised me to have a clinical study done and to publish the results. Dr. Steinbrocker referred me for this purpose to St. Vincent's Hospital in New York City, where Dr. Samuel Sverdlik, head of the rehabilitation department, supervised a clinical study of twenty-three carefully screened arthritis patients—eighteen with rheumatoid arthritis and five with osteoarthritis. Six to eight months passed between the time the patients applied for the study and the time the study was started. This represented a control period during which their hand disabilities continued and no Hand Gym exercises were done. After this, the patients embarked on a four-month program of twice-daily exercising with the Hand Gym. At the beginning and at monthly intervals, the chief occupational therapist at St. Vincent's, Anita Simmons, took strength and flexibility measurements and checked the patients' ability to do certain functional jobs like turning a key in a lock, opening a jar, and picking up small objects. The supervising physician, Dr. Judith Schauffler, saw the patients on the same days and evaluated their progress. At the end of the study, the majority of the rheumatoid arthritis patients and all of the other arthritis patients exhibited increased flexibility and strength as well as improvement in their function. Several could close their fists completely, which they could not do before. They were able once again to hold eating utensils of regular design rather than the type with built-up handles which are used by many arthritics.

I am grateful for the twelve years of reasonably normal use of my hands that I have had since developing the Hand Gym and I look forward to continued functioning. I am also convinced that if I had started this exercise system much earlier during my arthritis, my hands would have been better protected and would be less deformed than they are today. I believe that such exercises help to educate the hand to function in a protective position, which minimizes the stress on joints. If this protective position is carried over from exercise sessions into daily life, joints are less liable to suffer destruction.

THE GOAL IS JOINT PROTECTION

☐ The philosophy of *joint protection* is the mainstay of physical and occupational therapy for the arthritic hand. The most important elements of joint protection are:

1. Educating the hand to function in a position that places minimal stress on the joints
2. Exercising to keep fingers flexible and strong to maintain the favorable position
3. Splinting of the hand to reduce inflammation and, if necessary, to prevent positions that produce deformity

Please note, however, that hand exercises are not intended to strengthen the hand to the point where it becomes capable of destroying its own joints in use. The clinical study showed that in rheumatoid arthritics, strengthening occurs to the highest degree in those fingers or in those particular muscles that have lost most of their strength. Thus a proper balance is reestablished.

As clinical studies have shown, strengthening exercises have to be done daily only for a period of a few months, and after that, only when the need for them is felt, but at least once weekly. Range-of-motion exercises, to maintain or increase flexibility, should be done daily, however.

ANATOMY OF THE HAND

☐ Before proceeding to describe the exercises, it will be helpful to study the following drawings of the hand to familiarize ourselves with the anatomical names of the various bones and joints (figs. 2, 2a). Occupational therapists who deal with arthritics try to teach these terms to their patients since it makes for easier communication about such matters as bones, joints, deformities, protective positions, exercise positions, and so forth.

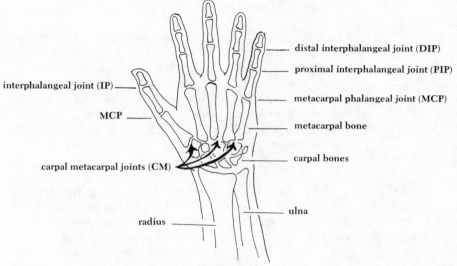

distal interphalangeal joint (DIP)

proximal interphalangeal joint (PIP)

interphalangeal joint (IP)

metacarpal phalangeal joint (MCP)

MCP

metacarpal bone

carpal bones

carpal metacarpal joints (CM)

ulna

radius

2. *Anatomical names for joints and bones of the hands*

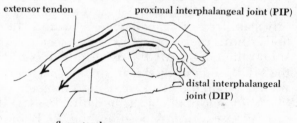

extensor tendon

proximal interphalangeal joint (PIP)

distal interphalangeal joint (DIP)

flexor tendon

2a. *Function of hand joints when grasping an object between the tip of the finger and the thumb*

TESTING THE HAND AND WRIST RANGES

□ First, let us test your fingers and hands for flexibility. These are the types of tests my rheumatologist asks me to perform during my biannual check-ups. If any of the ranges are limited, it is important to try to regain them by daily exercise.

Testing hand and wrist ranges, figures 3–14

• Spread fingers of both hands far apart (fig. 3). The fingers have to be straight. If you are at the point in your arthritis where you cannot straighten your fingers, use a support such as the edge of a table or the Hand Gym.

3. *Spread fingers as far apart as possible.*

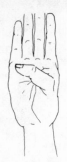

4. *Touch tip of thumb to base of little finger.*

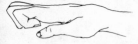

5. *Curl fingers so that tips touch the base of the fingers. Keep the large knuckles straight.*

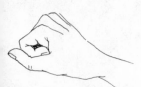

6. *Making a fist*

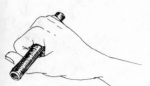

7. *Incorrect position for grasping: the MCP joint should not be bent.*

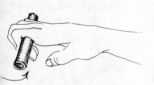

8. *Correct protective position for grasping objects: extend MCP and PIP; flex DIP.*

- Touch the tip of the thumb to the base of the little finger (fig. 4). If you cannot quite do this, rotate and circle the thumb a few times to warm it, then try again.
- Curl fingers so that tips of fingers touch the base of the fingers with the MCP (big knuckles) straight (fig. 5). If you cannot manage this, practice the exercise with the Hand Gym (figs. 20, 21). Finger-curling without and with resistance will help. This is an important test. If you cannot do it properly, it means that a very disabling finger deformity, the *swan-neck* deformity (fig. 16), could be in the process of forming.

Until recently, physicians merely wanted you to show that you could make a fist (fig. 6), but this is not a sufficient test of your flexibility. Also, please do not consider making a fist an adequate exercise; it does not stretch certain very important small muscles.

When the MCP joint is flexed, a large amount of muscle power is concentrated to pull the proximal phalanx into flexion. This could produce subluxation (partial dislocation) of the joint if the joint is not properly stabilized by its collateral ligaments. In rheumatoid arthritis these ligaments are subject to stretch, and subluxation of the MCP joint results. It is bad to bend the MCP joint during the grasp (fig. 7). That is why we want to "train the hand" in using a protective position (fig. 8) for grasping objects in daily life as well as during exercises. In this position, the MCP joint is kept extended and the PIP and DIP joints are flexed. (PIP are small joints in the middle of the finger; DIP are small joints near the fingertips.)

If you cannot make a fist, don't force it. It could do harm by placing undue stress on the ligaments of the MCP joints. Instead, exercise as shown in figure 21 to keep fingers flexible.

The ranges of motion of the wrists usually are evaluated at the same time as the fingers. A full range of wrist motion is important for two reasons. First, the muscles whose tendons span the wrists are placed under slight stretch as the wrist is articulated. The finger flexors are stretched when the wrist is extended (fig. 10) and the finger extensors when the wrist is flexed (fig. 11). This slight stretch makes the muscle more efficient. Similar considerations hold true for the other motions of the wrists.

Wednesday Night: Hands and Wrists

9. *Turn both hands out (abduct) and in (adduct).*

10. *Extend both wrists, upward.*

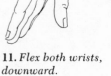

Second, the various motions of the wrists are necessary in everyday life. They come into play when we are shaving, brushing our teeth, stirring a pot, bathing, putting on clothes. Restricted motion of the wrist is very hampering.

Test the wrist ranges in the following way:

- Abduct both wrists by turning them out. Adduct both wrists by turning them inward (fig. 9). Extend both wrists all the way by turning them up (fig. 10) and flex both wrists by turning them all the way down (fig. 11).

  The drawings show the limits of the ranges that should be obtained. If you exercise and don't reach these limits, move slowly, and tighten your wrist muscles for about two seconds, relax, and turn further (figs. 9, 10, 11).
- Rotate the wrists (fig. 12).

  During evaluation of this exercise, note whether you develop any pain in describing the largest circle possible. If you are, stop just before the point of pain, contract the muscles, relax, and circle once or twice again.
- *Pronate* the hands by rotating the forearms and wrists so that the palms of the hands are down. Then *supinate* the hands so that the palms of the hands are up (fig. 13).

11. *Flex both wrists, downward.*

12. *Rotate both wrists in the largest circle possible. Circle in both directions.*

13. *Pronate and supinate the hands, by turning hands and forearm together, in and out.*

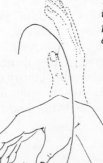

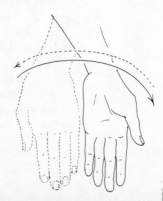

HAND DEFORMITIES

14. *Correct protective position for grasping objects: extend MCP and PIP; flex DIP.*

□ If the following discussion of hand deformities seems to you too complex to go into at this point, you can skip it and proceed with the description of Hand Gym exercises. Knowledge of the kinesiology, or function, of the hand and of deformities is not necessary in order to carry out exercises properly, but some readers may be interested in the subject.

Everybody, however, should be fully aware of the importance of the protective position of the hand (fig. 14), which is used in the Hand Gym exercises, and then carried over into daily life.

In the normal use of the hand—that is, the way the hand is used by a normal person without disabilities —the phalanges are usually first moved into a position so that they clear the object to be grasped. This means the hand is opened sufficiently to accommodate the object. Next, the fingers are bent to conform to the surface of the object to be grasped. Finally the object is grasped and held. The motions of the fingers and individual phalanges involved are flexion, extension, abduction, adduction, and rotation.

The fingers are moved by *extrinsic* and *intrinsic* hand muscles. The powerful extrinsics are located in the forearm and send their tendons through the wrist to attach to the various phalanges. When you hold your hand over your knee, and press into the knee with your fingertips or with the middle phalanges, you can feel, by touching the lower part of your forearm, how the flexor muscles bulge as you exert pressure on your knee. When you straighten out your hand against the underside of a table, for instance, you can feel the extrinsic extensor muscles in the back of your forearm; these are the antagonists to the much stronger flexors.

The intrinsic muscles are located within the hand itself. Most of them are hard to detect as they are located right between the bones. They are called *interossei* (meaning "between bones"). Together with the extrinsic extensors, they help to abduct, adduct, and rotate the fingers. One of the interossei, the very important dorsal interosseus no. 1, can be observed between the roots of the index finger and the thumb. When you abduct the index finger strongly against resistance you can feel the belly of this muscle contracting, if you touch it with a fingertip of the other hand.

Ulnar Deviation

The interosseus no. 1 is a very important muscle. It keeps the index finger from slipping into the ulnar direction (that is the direction away from the thumb and toward the ulna, the outer bone of the forearm) when pressure is placed on the side of the index finger, as in turning a key in a lock. This immediately gives us an idea of where the common *ulnar deviation* deformity comes from. (In figure 15, all fingers, not only the index finger, are deviating in the direction of the ulna.) A hand-rest splint helps to control it (fig. 15a).

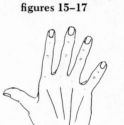

15. *Ulnar deviation*

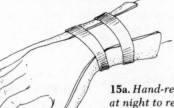

15a. *Hand-rest splint. Wear it at night to reduce inflammation and to control ulnar deviation if present.*

As long as fingers remain flexible, this ulnar deviation does not present much of a handicap, except that you lose the ability to oppose the tips of the little finger and the thumb. It results in a slight decrease of dexterity of which many old people, even those without arthritis, complain. However, once you permit your fingers to become stiff in those positions of deformity, they are liable to become nonfunctional. The difficulty with this deformity and with subluxation (see below) is that if the condition goes untreated it will prevent you from flattening out your hand, so that you have difficulty in opening the hand sufficiently to grasp large objects. And once you lose the ability to grasp, your hand quickly becomes weaker and stiffer just by disuse. It is very important to keep the hands flexible so that these two types of deformities, namely ulnar deviation and the subluxation of the MCP joints, do not interfere with your function.

My hands, after fifteen years of arthritis, show both of these conditions in a pronounced way; however, my fingers are very flexible, and although my hands are not as strong as they used to be, I can carry out practically all functions. I do make use of two devices that permit me to get better leverage and so reduce the strain on my finger joints. These are a key holder and a jar opener available at surgical supply stores. (See Directory of Aids, chapter 8.)

I am dismayed to read exercise instructions for arthritic hands that call for repeated turning of keys in locks and opening of jars to strengthen fingers. I can state from my own experience that as you lose the power to turn a key in a lock or to open a jar, you automatically want to repeat these motions again and again in order not to lose those functions. This same holds true, for instance, for making a fist. However, the results are miserable. The painful joints which produce the weakness in the first place become even more painful. Such exercises it seems to me, don't take into account the causes of pain, particularly joint misalignment and muscle imbalance.

Deliberate isometric exercises for the individual muscle in positions in which the joints are supported and protected, as in the Hand Gym, produce the desired results. I noticed this myself after a few months' use of the Hand Gym; it was also observed with most patients in the Hand Gym study who had these functional complaints. It seems paradoxical that once the strength has been regained to the point where you can use a key or unscrew a jar, you should still use mechanical devices to help you with these functions. The reason is that you want to place a minimum amount of stress on your joints in order to preserve them. The additional strength obtained in the exercises here is useful first to stretch tight intrinsic muscles through finger-curling, and second, to create muscle balance around the various finger joints so that any pressure in any direction on the fingers will be distributed uniformly and produce a minimum of stress on ligaments which are weakened through disease.

This principle can be graphically illustrated in connection with quadriceps muscles of the thigh. When I developed difficulty in climbing stairs, my therapist told me to strengthen the quadriceps muscles. These muscles, which extend the knee, had become very weak after several months of bed rest due to an illness not connected with arthritis. Before I consulted the therapist, I tried to force myself to climb stairs but was severely limited in this by pain in my knees. This pain was not necessarily arthritic pain. It was probably from undue strain on ligaments that were called upon to stabilize the knee in the absence of sufficiently strong muscle power. After two weeks of concentrated quadriceps muscles exercises, my stair-climbing became very easy and the knee pain was gone. Some of my readers who may have already observed the need for quadriceps exercise will be able to transfer the principle behind the knee exercises to finger exercises; namely, that strengthening muscles around joints stabilizes the joints, reduces joint pain by making it possible to use the joints more efficiently, and improves function.

Swan-Neck Deformity

In the very disabling deformity called *swan neck*, the middle phalanx rides up instead of continuing in a straight line with the proximal phalanx. The distal phalanx is flexed but cannot grip objects (fig. 16). A splint to control the deformity is shown in figure 16a. Among the factors contributing to this deformity is the abnormal pull (contracture) of intrinsic muscles, which prevents you from curling the fingers as indicated in figure 8, with the MCP joints (big knuckles) straight. Eventually, the middle phalanx cannot be flexed at all, and if there is some damage to the structure around the PIP joint, the middle phalanx will ride up in an abnormal way. The distal phalanx will flex automatically due to abnormal tendon pull, but the unnatural position of the proximal phalanx makes it impossible to grasp anything with this flexed distal phalanx. The finger will eventually become stiff from disuse in this abnormal position.

Subluxation of the MCP joint (fig. 16b) is another contributing factor in the swan-neck deformity. Subluxation takes place when a joint is properly aligned when extended, but improperly aligned when *flexed*. This subluxation displaces the tendon of the intrinsic muscles in such a way as to produce an effect similar to muscle contracture (shortening). The muscle is not shortened, but the tendon has to reach around the subluxed base of the proximal phalanx, so that there is not enough slack for the tendons to bend around the proximal phalanx. Although my right hand is severely subluxed, I was able to keep the proximal phalanx flexible enough through exercise of the type shown in figure 21 that I could continue to use the protective position.

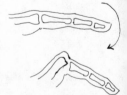

16. *Swan-neck deformity*

16a. *Swan-neck ring—a splint to help finger bend properly.*

16b. *Subluxation of the big knuckles can contribute to swan-neck deformity.*

Loss of ability to curl the fingers at the PIP joint means that the arthritic cannot grasp objects like flatware. I have used regular flatware during my fifteen years of arthritis, which I think is remarkable considering that thirteen years ago, before I exercised them properly, my fingers had started to stiffen at wrong angles so that I could hardly grasp anything. The PIP joints of several fingers of my left hand were so far destroyed that the joint spaces practically disappeared, as observed on the X-ray. Joint space is the distance between the bones where they come together in the joint. Normally the joint space is filled up by the cartilage, which covers the ends of both bones. It is not seen in X-rays because it does not contain the calcium of which bone is made and which is seen in the X-ray. Thus, when no joint space is seen, the cartilage must have disappeared.

I later developed ankyloses in several of the PIP joints. This can happen either by the bones growing together (bony ankylosis) or by fibers forming across the joint to stiffen it (fibrous ankylosis). The stiffness itself is disagreeable, as bumping into objects with the stiff finger is likely to produce pain. It is worse if the joint ankyloses at the wrong angle so that the finger becomes useless.

While the joints were still flexible, I had some functional splints made, the so-called swan-neck rings shown in figure 16a. (A functional splint is designed to allow you to perform tasks and not for complete immobilization.) The swan-neck rings are double rings connected at one point and made to fit snugly, so that the finger is forced into as normal a position as possible. Wearing these rings, I was able to use my left hand for grasping because the middle phalanges were supported in the bent position and the distal phalanges could flex freely. Eventually, several PIP joints on the left hand ankylosed in a functional position and I did not have to wear the swan-neck rings anymore. My left hand remained functional, although in a limited way. Some fingers were able to wrap around relatively large objects.

Metal swan-neck rings (preferable to plastic rings, since they are thin and therefore interfere less with grasping) usually are made in the orthotics departments of hospitals or at rehabilitation institutes. Once the swan-neck deformity is fixed, with the phalanges stiffened at wrong angles, the only correction I know

of is joint-replacement surgery. Such surgery uses
plastic implants in the joints. Some flexibility of joints
is regained and—to a very limited degree—some
strength as well.

Boutonniere Deformity

In this deformity (fig. 17), the middle phalanx is per-
manently flexed and the distal phalanx hyperextended. Objects cannot be gripped because of the bent
position of the middle phalanx. This deformity comes
about through damage to the tendinous structure on
both sides of the PIP joint as a result of inflammation
and swelling of the joint. A tear in this structure occurs, which prevents the middle phalanx from being
extended. The main therapy is prevention. Because
this deformity is due to inflammation of the PIP joint,
manifesting itself through profuse swelling, the inflammation and swelling have to be combatted, mainly
by resting the joint by immobilizing it in a short splint.
The damage to the joint proceeds very slowly, and
immobilizing it, which preferably should be done by
an occupational therapist, is very effective.

17. Boutonniere deformity. This requires preventive splinting.

One hand condition which is not called a deformity,
but which I found very disabling, is the inability to
make a fist. For instance, when I could not touch the
palm of my hand with my fingertips, I had difficulty
holding down the sleeve of a jacket when I put on an
overcoat. Even such small disabilities produce great
frustrations. I was gratified, then, to find out that after
a week or two of daily finger-curling (fig. 21) my hand
felt looser, and that shortly thereafter I could again
make a complete fist. I realized that I could overcome
a progressive deforming process and keep the PIP
joints flexible.

HAND-REST SPLINTING

☐ As I mentioned before, resting a joint helps to reduce the swelling and inflammation. The trouble with
hands is that even if you rest in bed, the phalanges of
the fingers are still likely to move, either for no appar-
ent reason or, for instance, in pulling up the bedcover
or in supporting your body when you roll over on your
side. This is enough movement to prevent the joint

from being sufficiently rested to reduce inflammation. Therefore, a rest splint is indicated if you want to reduce inflammation in all joints of the hands. Such a splint (fig. 15a) gives complete rest to all finger joints as well as to the wrist. A molded plastic shell is available, which can be adjusted to fit individual hands. It is individually fitted by an occupational therapist on prescription by a physician.

I have found these splints very beneficial, especially when worn at night during periods of high disease activity. When I wore the splint on one hand and not on the other, I could really notice the difference the next morning. When I consider that this simple mechanical means produced unswelling of my red, hot knuckles—something which twelve aspirin a day could not achieve and which cortisone injections into the joints could only temporarily achieve—I am very impressed by the performance of rest splints.

Hand-rest splinting is not very popular, possibly because the rheumatologist, and especially the general practitioner, may be at a loss to advise you where to get such a splint. After my rheumatologist told me to get one, I went through several frustrating experiences until I finally found a hospital with an occupational therapist who could fit me with splints. The therapist told me she had very little call for them.

FUNCTIONAL SPLINTS

☐ There are also functional splints available in addition to the swan-neck ring described earlier, which I found to be the easiest of all the functional splints to tolerate. Another very useful splint is used to correct thumb deformity. In the usual thumb deformity, the proximal phalanx is bent and the distal phalanx is hyperextended to compensate for the flexed MCP joint. In this position the thumb can exert only a very small force. Without splinting or surgical intervention, the thumb becomes useless.

I tried a variety of functional splints for my thumb which would keep the MCP joint in extension and permit flexion of the PIP joint. Most of them were unpleasant to wear, as they prevented rotation of the thumb to oppose the various fingers. After some research I found that the Warm Springs Foundation, Warm Springs, Georgia, had designed a slim metal splint which suited my condition and which permitted opposition of the thumb. To my surprise, I could not get this duplicated at any of the major rehabilitation and hospital centers in New York. Finally, the orthotics department of the Institute of Rehabilitation Medicine, New York University Medical Center, reproduced the design in plastic. I have worn this splint on my right hand for approximately eleven years. I wore a similar splint on my left hand for eight years and found to my delight that I could discontinue using it, as the fibers around my MCP joint have regenerated, making use of the splint unnecessary.

Splinting is worth trying for the thumb, but there are also some sophisticated surgical procedures available, in which tendons are rerouted across the MCP joints of the thumb to bring it back into extension. It is advisable to look carefully for a surgeon who is experienced in this type of delicate surgery, however.

There are several other functional hand splints. Those designed to keep the proximal phalanges extended, or to prevent ulnar deviation of the fingers, are among the most useful. Several designs of such splints are known to occupational therapists. It is important to have these splints fitted individually. They tend to create pressure points around the large knuckles and to be clumsy, since they usually cover at least part of the palm. The prospect of having to wear such splints gives me a powerful incentive to exercise my fingers instead. However, when hands are inflamed, such splints can be useful in supporting the fingers in the correct position and preventing you from doing too much work and thereby increasing your discomfort.

THE HAND GYM SYSTEM

☐ We now turn to the exercises for the Hand Gym. (Catalog number F70900, Maddak, Inc., Pequannock, N.J. 07440. Available through selected surgical supply stores, Sears, Roebuck, or the manufacturer, at twenty dollars.) As I mentioned earlier, a clinical study of eighteen patients with rheumatoid arthritis and five patients with osteoarthritis produced statistically significant increases in strength and range of motion in those patients who had exercised twice a day for four months. Most patients reported improved function. A follow-up after four years showed that these patients had continued to exercise without supervision on the average of once a week, and more than half of the rheumatoid arthritis patients had retained their improvement of function gained during the four-month study. All of the osteoarthritis patients had maintained their functional improvements.

I myself noticed a definite improvement in my function after about two weeks of exercising daily. I have been able to improve my handwriting at various times in the last twelve years, at times when I was dissatisfied with it, by exercising several times daily for a few days.

The Hand Gym is supplied with a thirty-page instruction booklet and a large exercise chart with drawings and photographs. The booklet contains detailed descriptions of seven range-of-motion exercises for the fingers and wrist and thirteen isometric strengthening exercises for the fingers, indicating also the anatomical names of the muscles.

The exercises are considered a highly efficient means to maintain and increase range of motion and strength—not only for arthritics but also for persons without arthritis whose hands have stiffened with age, and for persons to whom manual dexterity is important, such as musicians, dentists, typists, and precision assemblers.

Persons with rheumatoid arthritis or an injury to the hand(s) require a balanced medical treatment program, of which the Hand Gym exercises form but one important part. The Hand Gym is an exercise aid; *no one with rheumatoid arthritis or injury should use it without initial professional instruction and supervision by a physician or therapist.*

The stretching exercises help to increase and maintain the ranges of motion. The isometric exercises strengthen the hand muscles through the production of a *brief, maximal* effort of each muscle against resistance with the least amount of stress on the joints.

One five-minute session each day will help you regain or maintain agility and strength in your hands and fingers. Several sessions each day will help you to regain elasticity of tightened muscles, and to develop endurance.

Please note that gripping exercises should be avoided with those fingers that have excessive pain, joint swelling, or inflammatory tenderness in the second finger joints (PIP). This condition should be reported to your physician to enable further treatment and resumption of exercise.

THE DAILY FIVE-MINUTE WORKOUT WITH THE HAND GYM

☐ Hold the Hand Gym flat against your body at waist level with elbows against your sides. You may be sitting, standing, or lying down. The "Hand Gym" name should face upward.

In the basic exercise position for many exercises, rest your palms flat against the sides of the Hand Gym so that roots of your fingers lie against the foam cushions. Insert your fingers into the proper slots. Let your thumbs rest on the upper surface. Do each exercise with both hands simultaneously.

To help prevent finger deformities and minimize pain, use the *protective position* for the rheumatoid hands (fig. 18):

Five-minute workout with the Hand Gym, figures 18–32

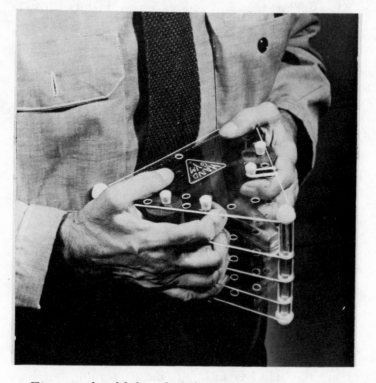

18. *Exercising with the Hand Gym. Fingers in "protective position."*

Fingers should be slightly spread, large knuckle joint "K" should be kept straight, and small joints should be bent slightly. In this position your fingers are supported, joints are properly lined up, and pain is minimized. According to present medical opinion, deformities can be prevented or reduced if the hand is held in this "protective position" during exercises and when grasping things in daily activities.

In closing your hand when grasping, it is harmful to bend the big knuckle joint, since this puts stress on that joint and contributes to deforming the hand by stretching the ligaments. Use of the Hand Gym encourages the correct position.

If there is swelling or pain in the middle joint of any finger, omit exercises for this finger until it is improved. Consult your doctor.

Finger Spreading Without Resistance

19. *Finger spreading without resistance (with or without Gym).*

• If your hands are normal do this without the Hand Gym. However, if you have arthritis or other hand problems, use the Hand Gym for support. Rest your palms against the Gym and leave your fingers "floating" free outside the slots (fig. 19).

Spread fingers as far apart as you can, then press them tightly together. Repeat four times. Now spread fingers apart and move middle finger up toward index finger, and then down toward ring finger. Repeat four times.

Be sure that you do not omit moving the middle finger—separately—toward the index finger and again toward the ring finger. This may not be easy at first, but you will succeed after a while. I have observed that with many people—even musicians, whose fingers could be expected to be very nimble—the middle finger is the first one to exhibit stiffness.

If you require support for your fingers in order to flatten the hand, and you want to exercise in the course of the day when you do not have the Hand Gym available, you may perform the exercise while pressing the palms of your hands near the roots of your fingers against the edge of a table.

Finger-Spreading with Resistance

• Hold the Hand Gym in the basic position, but let fingers rest against exercise bar (in second hole above foam cushions).

Spread fingers apart, pressing as hard as possible outward against walls of the Hand Gym (fig. 19a). Hold to a count of six. Now bring fingers together, pressing as hard as possible inward against walls (fig. 19b). Hold to a count of six. Press middle finger against one wall and hold to a count of six; then press it against opposite wall and hold to a count of six (fig. 19c). Then do the same with each of the other fingers.

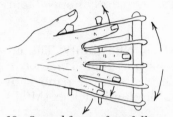

19a. Spread fingers forcefully outward against the walls of the Gym for a count of six.

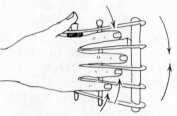

19b. Bring fingers together against the walls of the Gym forcefully for the count of six.

19c. Press middle finger strongly against one wall for a count of six, then against the opposite wall.

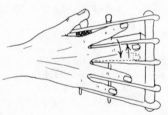

This, together with finger-curling with resistance, is one of the most important exercises on the Hand Gym. The Hand Gym structure works here to advantage, and cannot be easily replaced by other objects in the household. When you place your fingers in the slots and spread them against the walls, you will become aware of the strength with which each finger can press against the one side or the other side. You will then also notice that some fingers may be weaker than others, especially when pushed in one or the other direction. This should give you an incentive to exercise the weaker finger diligently in order to achieve a good balance of strength. The abduction and adduction of the fingers are accomplished by the interossei muscles which help rotate the finger, as when grasping a pencil, an eating utensil, or a hammer.

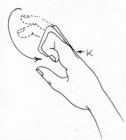

20. *Start with fingers straight. Slowly curl fingers, keeping large knuckles "K" straight, four times briefly. If you cannot touch fingertips to palm with large knuckles straight, practice next exercise with the Hand Gym.*

Finger-Curling Without Resistance

• If your hands are normal, do this without the Hand Gym (fig. 20). However, if you have arthritis or other hand problems, use the Hand Gym for support.

  Start with fingers straight. Then curl fingers into a hook; it is very important to keep knuckle joint "K" straight while doing this. Continue curling as hard as possible until fingertips touch palms. Repeat four times.

  This is an exercise to test your flexibility. The arthritic often will require the support of the Hand Gym and will usually not be able to touch the palm with the fingertips while keeping the big knuckles (MCP) straight.

Finger-Curling with Resistance

• Hook fingers around foam cushions and squeeze briefly four times, as hard as possible each time, *keeping knuckle joint "K" straight* (fig. 21).

21. *Curl fingers forcefully around foam rubber four times. Keep big knuckles "K" straight.*

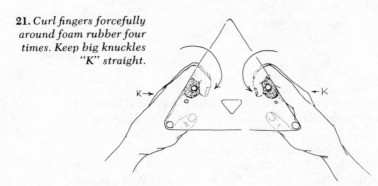

  This is an important exercise to keep the fingers flexible and to loosen the intrinsic muscles and thereby counteract the disabling swan-neck deformity. Squeezing briefly four times should not produce any pain. It it does, or if the middle joint of a finger (PIP) is inflamed, swollen, or painful, omit this exercise until the finger is recovered. Consult your physician.

Two Exercises for Finger-Straightening with Resistance

- Place exercise bars in second holes above cushions, away from the edge, and stretch rubber bands across the ends of the bars.
- For the first exercise, insert fingers in slots between rubber band and exercise bar so that rubber band is stretched across lower part of fingers above big knuckle joints (fig. 22). Push each finger (the same finger of each hand together) as hard as possible outward against the rubber band. Hold to a count of six each time.

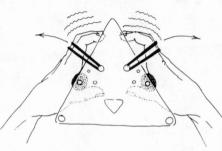

22. Push fingers of both hands outward against rubber band, hold to a count of six. If you can, exercise each finger separately.

- For the second exercise, pull fingers out far enough so that upper part of fingers rest against the rubber band. Then push each finger outward against the rubber band, as hard as possible. Do this with one finger of each hand at a time. Hold to a count of six each time (fig. 23).

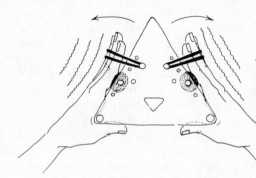

23. Slip hands down so middle joint rests on foam rubber. Push forefinger out against rubber band for a count of six. If you can, exercise each finger separately.

The extrinsic extensor muscle is strengthened in the first exercise. It helps to keep fingers straight and acts together with the interossei muscles to rotate the fingers.

In the second exercise, the lumbricalis muscle is strengthened. This muscle helps to straighten the forepart of each finger and helps to control the pinch between tips of fingers and thumb. It also controls the strength of tapping, such as in typing or piano-playing, by acting as a brake on the profundus muscle, which bends the fingertip.

Finger-Bending, Distal Phalanx

• Place exercise bar in second hole above foam cushions, away from edge, and stretch rubber band across ends of bar, as shown in figure 24.

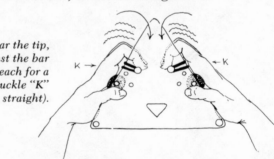

24. *Press fingers near the tip, one at a time, against the bar as hard as possible, each for a count of six (large knuckle "K" straight).*

Place fingers in slots just far enough so that fingertips can rest on bar. Keeping knuckle joint "K" straight, press one finger, *near the tip*, at a time against the bar *as hard as possible*. Hold to a count of six each time.

This exercise strengthens the profundus muscle, which is located in the forearm and sends its tendon all the way out to the fingertip to bend it. This, as well as the next exercise, is only safe for the rheumatoid arthritic if he can flatten out his hand so that the MCP joint, big knuckle (K), is kept straight during the exercise. I recommend that persons who cannot flatten their hands against the top of the bed should not use the Hand Gym, since they will be unable to assume the protective position, which safeguards the big knuckle, during exercises. They should work with a therapist to loosen their hands first, if possible, and to straighten them sufficiently to fit the Hand Gym.

Finger-Bending, Middle Phalanx

• Place exercise bar in second hole above foam cushions, close to the edge.

Press *middle* section of each finger, one at a time, against the bar *as hard as possible.* Hold to count of six each time. Remember to keep knuckle joint "K" straight (fig. 25).

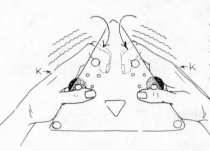

25. *Press middle section of one finger at a time against the bar as hard as possible, for a count of six. (Note that bar is moved for this exercise to second hole above foam rubber. Large knuckle "K" straight).*

This exercise strengthens the sublimis (also called superficialis) muscle, which is located in the forearm and whose tendon leads into the hand to bend the middle joint (PIP) of the fingers. This is the principal muscle used in carrying heavy loads such as suitcases or in gripping tightly—around the handle of a hammer, for instance.

Sideways Thumb Movement (Up)

• Pull each cushioned hand rest bar out one-half inch. Holding the Hand Gym in the basic position, push thumbs *up* against the protruding bars as hard as possible. Hold to a count of six (fig. 26).

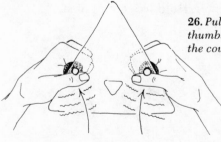

26. *Pull exercise bar out a little. Press thumbs forcefully* up *against bar to the count of six.*

Sideways Thumb Movement (Down)

- Keep cushioned hand rest bars pulled out one-half inch. Press thumbs *down* as hard as possible against protruding bars (fig. 27). Hold to a count of six.

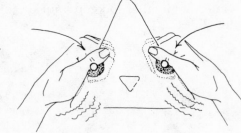

27. *Press thumbs forcefully down against exercise bar for a count of six.*

Thumb-Flexing (with Thumb Straight)

- Keeping thumbs *straight,* push in against the ends of the hand rest bars with each thumb, as hard as possible (fig. 28). Continue pushing and hold to a count of six.

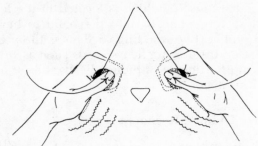

28. *With straight thumbs, press against bar ends firmly for a count of six.*

Flexing, Tip of Thumb

- Hold the Hand Gym in the basic position. Press the *tip* of each thumb as hard as possible against the front wall (fig. 29). Hold to a count of six.

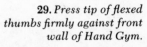

29. *Press tip of flexed thumbs firmly against front wall of Hand Gym.*

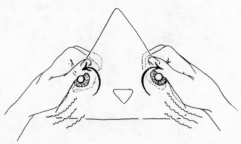

Thumb-Straightening, Proximal Phalanx

• Curl your left fingers around the top of the Hand
Gym. Place left thumb between first and second
walls. Now bend thumb at small joint, pressing the
joint as hard as possible against front wall (fig. 30).
Hold to a count of six. Repeat with right thumb.

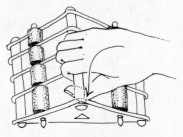

30. *Press thumb joint outward against Hand Gym's inner front wall. Hold for a count of six. Repeat with other hand.*

Thumb-Straightening, Distal Phalanx

• Proceed as in last exercise, but this time press the
nail of each thumb against the outside wall as hard
as possible (fig. 31). Hold to a count of six each time.

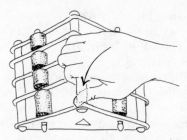

31. *Assume the same hand position, but press the thumbnail outward for a count of six.*

Thumb Rotation

With index fingers and thumbs lying flat on outer wall,
"roll" your thumbs along the surface of the wall toward you, then press them against wall as hard as possible (fig. 32). Hold to a count of six. If you prefer, do
this one thumb at a time.

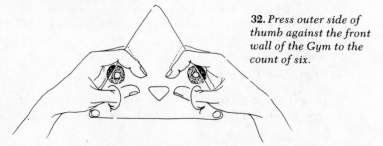

32. *Press outer side of thumb against the front wall of the Gym to the count of six.*

The preceding seven exercises show various directions in which the thumb is pressed up and down, flexed and extended, and finally rotated. Individual muscles usually are responsible for obtaining these motions. The bellies of these muscles can be felt in the palm, near the root of the thumb, and form what is called the thenar eminence. As you give resistance to the thumb, you can notice contraction of muscles within the thenar eminence. When you give resistance to the fingertip of the little finger, you will notice contraction of the hypothenar eminence on the palm at the root of the little finger. A rotating, or opponens, muscle of the little finger, similar to that of the thumb, exists also and can be exercised as shown in the Hand Gym exercise booklet.

It is important to keep the muscles of the thumb in shape. After all, the thumb represents half the hand in grasping, as objects are grasped between this finger and the other four. If you require a splint to straighten out the MCP joint of your thumb, wear it during the exercises, since the Hand Gym does not supply support for the MCP joint of the thumb, as it does for the other fingers.

After exercising for a few weeks, you will notice that as you grasp the thumb between the index finger and the thumb of the other hand and try to wiggle out of the pinch in various directions, your joints hurt less, being controlled now more by increased muscle power than by the ligaments, which may be weakened due to the disease and painful when stretched.

Thumb Rotation, the last exercise (fig. 32), is an isometric exercise to strengthen the opponens muscle of the thumb. However, it does not stretch the muscle; some stretching is achieved by the first exercise. Specific stretching of the opponens muscle is accomplished by resting the hand on a table and lifting the thumb up as high as possible.

Other physical treatment considerations for the hand, besides exercises, include: (1) balanced activity to protect joints, (2) heat and massage, and (3) splints and gloves.

Protecting the Joints

Hands must always be used, we cannot help that. If we can no longer use our hands, we are condemned to be helped even with eating, dressing, and body hygiene. I find it a very great incentive to avoid such handicaps. Therefore, it is of prime importance to maintain flexibility and sufficient strength to be able to operate within the condition dictated by the weakness of our joints. Even if you are able to handle a key or to open a screw jar, don't display false pride by unnecessarily performing these actions. Use a key holder and a jar opener to provide leverage. Use a protective position of the hand for grasping objects in daily life (fig. 8). Do not subject your hands to wear and tear; instead maintain strength and flexibility through exercises. The daily stretching and the weekly strengthening exercises are probably sufficient to accomplish this—unless you have just passed through an acute phase and are weak, in which case you may require daily strengthening of finger muscles for a while. Remember that strengthening your hands in the protective position with the Hand Gym is more efficient and less harmful than using your hands forcefully in activities like washing and wringing laundry.

Use mechanical aides such as electric washers and dryers whenever you can. A booklet prepared by Judith Klinger with the Institute of Rehabilitation Medicine, New York University Medical Center, and the Campbell Soup Company, called *Mealtime Manual for People with Disabilities and the Aging,* contains a host of good suggestions and descriptions of gadgets to reduce the strain in the kitchen. The Arthritis Foundation also publishes a booklet describing useful self-help devices *Self-Help Manual for Arthritic Patients* (see Directory of Aids). Select and try some of them to help you in those activities which seem stressful for your hands.

Heat Treatments

My rheumatologist suggested to me early in the disease to soak my hands for twenty minutes every morning in water as hot as I could stand, and after this to dry the hands and use an ointment such as Ben-Gay to lengthen the effect of increased circulation. Epsom salts can be added to the water.

I have found this treatment beneficial in those times when I suffered from knuckle inflammation and pain. However, this twenty-minute bath can be quite time-consuming. It takes time to set it up, and you may need to rest afterwards. I found that water hot enough to increase the circulation in my hands to the degree that they turned red produced perspiration in other parts of the body such as head, neck, and chest. To save time, I started soaking my hands in a small whirlpool bath with very hot water for five minutes. The massage produced by the water jet makes you more comfortable, permits the use of a higher water temperature, and helps in unswelling fingers slightly (fig. 33).

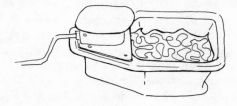

33. *A small Sears Roebuck whirlpool bath can be used for soaking hands.*

Splints and Gloves

Use of night rest splints or stretch gloves, or even both together as I have tried, helps to reduce inflammation and swelling of the whole finger. I often felt so comfortable wearing these aids at night that I only needed to wash my hands with soap and warm water in the morning to feel "in shape." Stretch gloves act like elastic bandages around each finger to force superfluous fluid out of them. They also cause the surface temperature to rise slightly, which is very pleasant. In the depths of winter, I wear a pair of fur-lined leather gloves. These keep my fingers warm and comfortable and also keep them in extension, though not quite as effectively as would a rest splint.

In chapter 4, "What to Do About Pain and Stiffness," I describe two other treatment modalities for the hands—mud packs and the paraffin wax dip. Both these treatments are supposed to offer a measure of relief from discomfort. I do not describe them here because I do not find them very effective for hands.

STRENGTHENING THE WRISTS

☐ Range-of-motion exercises for the wrists are shown in figures 9 and 12. Strengthening of the wrists can be accomplished by following exactly the range-of-motion exercises, but with resistance furnished by the other hand or by pressing in the prescribed directions against a part of your body, like the knee, or against a piece of furniture, like a tabletop or the arm of a chair.

HAND AWARENESS

☐ Once you have become accustomed to the various hand exercises and are aware of the function of various muscles, you may find it pleasant to incorporate some of the exercises into the motions of your daily life and to be aware of the stretching or strengthening these motions produce. For example, try several times a day to grasp a pencil between phalanges of your fingers with the MCP extended for a few seconds, as shown in figure 8.

At the slightest sign of developing tightness or loss of range or weakness, intensify your exercises by doing them more frequently. Clumsiness is not an inherent property, it can be largely cured by increasing the ranges of motion and strength of the fingers.

Note: For information about how you can obtain the devices and special equipment mentioned in this chapter, consult the Directory of Aids.

9 Thursday Night: Posture, Breathing, and Circulation

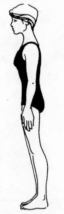

1. *Good posture— Stomach in, spine straight.*

□ I was one of the tallest boys in my class, so tall that the school desks were always too low for me. As a result, I got into the habit of curving my back when I sat in class, and this posture, unfortunately, carried over into my life outside school. My uncle, who was a physician, painted a dark picture of my future health if I did not straighten up, and fifty years later, after a few years of rheumatoid arthritis, I came to understand the wisdom of his concern. Because of my bad posture, I experienced pain in the muscles of my upper back which prevented me from sleeping properly for years, until the muscles were relaxed through heat treatments and exercise.

I remember the exercise my rheumatologist recommended for this upper back trouble. "Walk like a general for five minutes a day," he said. I was to keep my neck and back as straight as possible and my shoulders back (fig. 1). I tried this, but it was difficult to do and brought no improvement. Years later, though, I adapted a PNF (proprioceptive neuromuscular facilitation) exercise for the upper back and shoulders and had remarkable success. In as few as ten sessions, I was able to walk straight for the first time in more than forty years. I believe that in this case, only tightness of muscles was involved. The X-ray of my upper back

174

showed no arthritic changes, and fortunately, I did not suffer from ankylosing spondylitis, which can result in irreversible changes.

THE EFFECTS OF BAD POSTURE

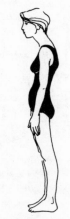

☐ Bad posture affects much more than a person's appearance. For example, a slouched forward posture causes the stomach to be pushed downward and out, which in turn hinders the diaphragm (the flat muscle dividing the chest and abdominal cavities) from pumping air out of the lungs (fig. 2). The lower (lumbar) spine curves to compensate for the curvature of the upper spine, and this can produce lower back pain. In the slouched position, the head is carried forward rather than upright. The neck muscles thus are not exercised through their full range, and stiffness and headaches result. Breathing is further impaired by a slouched or hunched posture, since the muscles across the front of the chest, the pectorals, tighten up and do not permit the rib cage to expand fully. All these consequences of poor posture can occur in a normal individual, especially with advancing age, and they explain a lot of the pain and discomfort experienced by the arthritic.

2. *Poor posture— Stomach out, neck bent.*

EXERCISES FOR BETTER POSTURE

☐ In a good posture, the spine is kept as straight as possible (fig. 1). Fortunately, this can be achieved by exercises to firm up the abdominal muscles, loosen the pectoral muscles, and strengthen the muscles of the upper back. This strengthening, together with loosening the neck muscles as described in chapter 6, will enable you to hold yourself erect, avoid the pain of bad posture, and breathe more easily.

There is one more important requirement for good posture. You must wear proper shoes, if necessary with corrective insoles (see chapter 11). Improper alignment of the feet, toeing in or out, can result in painful stresses on the knees or hips, and you may involuntarily respond to the pain by hunching your back. So, as an aid to good posture, be sure to wear comfortable shoes and have any problems of alignment corrected.

THE CHEST STRETCH

Loosening the pectorals, figures 3–7

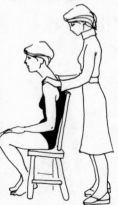

3. *Tense shoulders as if to move muscles forward.*

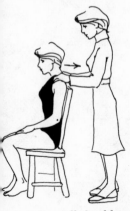

4. *Relax, roll shoulders back.*

□ • This exercise helps loosen the pectoral muscles. Sit on a high-backed chair; your therapist or helper will move your shoulders backward to straighten them as much as possible (fig. 3). When the limit is reached and the shoulders are being held tightly, strain against your helper's hands as strongly as possible by contracting the chest muscles to pull the shoulders forward. Do this for three seconds (count of six). Relax, and permit the shoulders to be moved gently backward by your therapist or helper (fig. 4). When you reach the limit, repeat the exercise. Do this several times, until no further improvement seems possible in that particular session.

• A second exercise to loosen the pectoral muscles is as follows: Sit on a high-backed chair, place your palms behind your head so that elbows stick out at right angles (fig. 5). Your therapist or helper pulls your elbows back as far as they can go without pain (fig. 6). At that point, push with your elbows against the helping hands as strongly as possible for three seconds (count of six). Relax. Permit your elbows to be gently moved backward as far as they can go without pain (fig. 7). Repeat the exercise until no further range is achieved.

Once you have achieved sufficient body awareness, you will be able to tense the pectoral muscles without straining against the hands of a helper. You will then be able to carry out both exercises—with your arms at your sides as well as with your hands behind your head—by yourself.

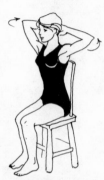

5. *Hands behind head, strain to move shoulders back.*

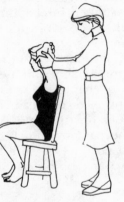

6. *Tense muscles as if to move elbows forward.*

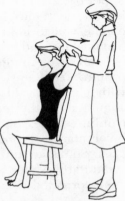

7. *Relax, move elbows back.*

STRENGTHENING THE UPPER BACK

• Still sitting on a high-backed chair, pull shoulder blades together as strongly as possible (fig. 8). Do this for six seconds (count of twelve). The more the pectoral muscles have been loosened in the earlier exercises, the easier it will be for you to bring your shoulder blades together.

• Next, still sitting on the chair, raise your right arm and move it back by contracting the back muscles as strongly as possible (fig. 9). Do this for three seconds (count of six).

Do the same exercise with your other arm.

• Now, do the above exercise with both arms, moving them back as far as possible by contracting the back muscles as strongly as possible (fig. 10). Do this for three seconds (count of six).

Strengthening the upper back, figures 8–12

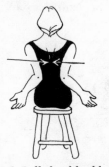 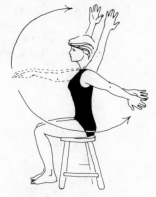

8. *Pull shoulder blades together to the count of six.*

9. *First one arm up to the count of six, then other arm up to the count of six.*

10. *Both arms up to the count of six.*

During the last three exercises, while you are raising the arms overhead and stretching the upper back muscles, keep your lower (lumbar) spine straight by pulling your stomach in.

Both the pectorals and the upper back benefit from the following movements, which you do while lying face down on the bed.

• Place a pillow at the middle of the bed and lie down with your stomach compressing the pillow; this helps straighten out your lower spine. Raise your right arm as high as possible (fig. 11). Hold position for three seconds (count of six). Lower the arm.

11. *Lift one arm up at a time.*

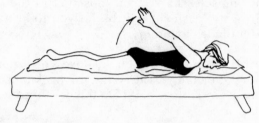

Repeat the exercise with your left arm. Raise the arm as high as possible for three seconds (count of six) and then lower it. If it is not too tiring, repeat the exercise several times with both arms, one at a time.

Finally, try to lift both arms simultaneously (fig. 12), even if you can only do it for a second or so. Gradually, with practice, you will notice that you can raise both arms simultaneously for a longer count. If you can raise both arms together for three seconds (count of six), you may discontinue the exercises in which one arm is raised at a time.

12. *Lift both arms up together.*

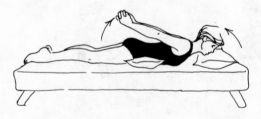

If you do not succeed in raising both arms, keep the arms at the side and try to raise your head and chest up from the bed. Do not use your arms and hands to help you in this exercise. If you do this movement repeatedly, it is isotonic. I prefer to do it isometrically, raising myself as high as possible for three to six seconds (count of six to twelve).

As you do these exercises a number of times, try to become aware of the muscle groups that are active. Eventually, you should be able occasionally to tense

the muscles that straighten your back and also those
that bring the shoulder blades together.

Avoid arching your lower back in the foregoing exercises. (The pillow under your stomach is an aid to
this. It helps to stabilize your lower back, and has the
same effect as contracting your abdominal muscles.)
We want to avoid arching the lower back, first, in order
to concentrate on strengthening the upper back in
these exercises, and second, in order not to aggravate
a possible dormant lower back problem.

LOOSENING THE UPPER BACK

☐ In the next two exercises we first tilt and then turn
the upper back.

• Sit on a chair and let your right arm hang down lower
  and lower at your side. Remain seated squarely on
  the chair and lower your arm slowly; only your upper
  back should tilt (fig. 13).

Repeat movement on the other side, letting the left
arm hang down.

• Curve your upper back forward, bending head down.
  Keep lower back straight (fig. 14).
  When you have resumed an upright position, contract your back muscles strongly for a count of six;
  this will produce a stretching as well as a strengthening effect. If you notice a certain stiffness in carrying out this exercise, repeat this and the next exercise
  several times.

**Curving the upper
back, figures 13 & 14**

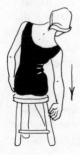

*13. Lower right arm
slowly as far as it will
go, then the other arm.*

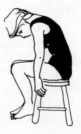

*14. Curve upper back
slowly down and up
again.*

• Sitting on a chair, rest your hands on your hips and slowly rotate your upper torso to the left as far as it will go (fig. 15). Do this gently. Then contract your back muscles as you rotate back to starting position. Now, rotate your upper body gently to the right as far as it will turn, then rotate slowly back to starting position, contracting your back muscles as you move (fig. 16).

Upper back rotation, figures 15 & 16

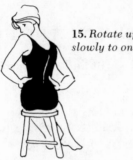

15. *Rotate upper back slowly to one side.*

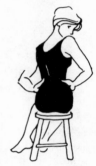

16. *Rotate to the other side.*

STRENGTHENING THE ABDOMEN FOR BACK SUPPORT

☐ This section deals with the abdominal muscles, which come into play both for good posture and easy breathing. When allowed to become slack, these muscles can no longer hold the intestines in place. As the intestines drop, they pull the spine out of its correct alignment.

If you have any problem with these exercises, discuss them with your doctor. If you have a protruding abdomen—perhaps following an operation or pregnancy, your doctor may prefer that you assist your posture and breathing at first by wearing an abdominal support and trying to do the sit-ups at a later time, after the abdomen has been contained.

Exercises for abdominal muscles usually are done while you are lying down on a firm flat surface or bed. They call for raising the upper part of your body to a sitting position while holding your knees slightly bent. If you are just beginning such exercises and have weak abdominal muscles, you will find them very hard to do; however, there are a number of variations that are easier to do at the beginning. Also at this stage you may need the help of someone to hold your feet down as you lift your upper body off the bed.

• The easiest way of doing the sit-ups is shown in figure 17. Sit at the edge of the bed. Slowly lean back and hold the position for two to three seconds. This is the easiest exercise to start with.

Sit-ups for abdominal strengthening, figures 17–21

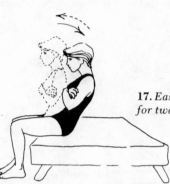

17. Easy does it. Lean back for two or three seconds.

A Slightly More Strenuous Sit-Up

• While lying on the bed, try to sit up while your legs are fully extended—knees straight (fig. 18). Be sure that the lumbar spine is flat on the bed and not hollow. If you cannot do this, have someone hold your feet down while you try to sit up. It is easier to do if your upper back and shoulders are resting on a pillow. If you don't have a helper to hold your feet down or otherwise assist you, a blanket wrapped around the mattress may provide the necessary anchor for your feet.

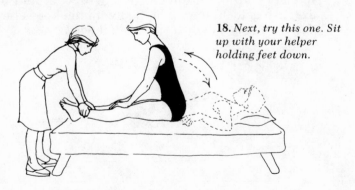

18. Next, try this one. Sit up with your helper holding feet down.

Sitting up with legs extended requires less effort, since the legs in this position provide a heavier counterbalance to the weight of the upper body that is being lifted. However, the lumbar spine is vulnerable in this position. When trying to sit up, you may actuate your hip flexors and thereby curve the lumbar spine in an inappropriate way (fig. 19). This can be dangerous for persons with lower back problems. When you are in the knees-up position (see figure 21), the lumbar spine remains flat on the bed as you sit up.

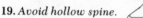
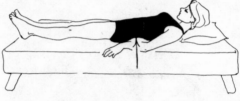

19. *Avoid hollow spine.*

It is important to go gradually from the easiest positions to the more difficult ones. Start with one you can do easily and repeat it a number of times. You will find out that after doing an easy exercise perhaps ten times, you will be able to do the next more difficult exercise two or three times, even on the same evening. Each time you exercise, try to step up to the next exercise on the scale of difficulty, provided it is suitable for you. The most effective exercises for the abdominal muscles are the following ones.

• Lie on your back on the bed with knees bent (fig. 20). Raise yourself from the lying-down position to the sitting position, keeping your knees bent. Lower yourself, raise yourself again, and try to repeat this sequence up to ten times. (A way to work into this exercise is to sit up on the bed with the knees bent, and then very slowly let yourself down.)

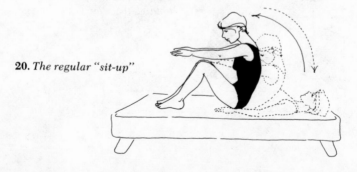

20. *The regular "sit-up"*

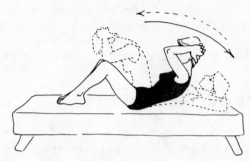

21. *With hands behind your head—more effective but more difficult.*

Finally, when you are strong enough, you should be able to do this exercise with your hands behind your head or your neck and knees bent (fig. 21). This shifts weight to the upper part of the body and makes the exercise a bit more difficult.

During the day you should be conscious of how you are holding your abdominal muscles; get accustomed to pulling your stomach in.

BREATHING

□ The importance of breathing and its mechanism was brought home to me only after I was struck by arthritis. This occurred very early in the disease when my rheumatologist explained to me that improved breathing would be helpful in combatting the extreme fatigue which accompanied my arthritis. Oxygen taken in when we breathe enters the blood by combining with hemoglobin, and is used in a process that helps to generate heat—mostly in the muscles—and to regenerate the cells of the body. If the available oxygen is reduced, these essential life processes become inefficient, and the body feels fatigued and seeks to rest, since during rest less oxygen is needed. In rheumatoid arthritis, the concentration of hemoglobin in the blood is generally reduced and thus there is less oxygen available.

Also, when the air is humid, our breathing apparatus has to work harder because our lungs are not only exchanging oxygen and carbon dioxide (the exhaust gas from our burning processes), but they are also taking on more work of eliminating extra moisture that, in drier conditions, would be eliminated to a large extent by evaporation from the skin.

Awareness of how our breathing apparatus functions will help us to understand the breathing exercises in this chapter. We will also learn how proper breathing helps the circulation and helps to keep us more fit.

THE MECHANICS OF BREATHING

☐ Breathing consists of inhaling and exhaling. The lungs are resilient, spongy organs that function somewhat like balloons. When we inhale they inflate; when we relax the muscles used in inhaling they deflate partially. And when we exhale deliberately they deflate further. Inhaling occurs when we enlarge the cavity enclosing the lungs; this has the effect of lowering air pressure within the lungs, causing air to enter from the outside in order to equalize the pressure. To enlarge the chest cavity, we can (1) expand the circumference of the rib cage by contracting the external intercostal muscles (muscles between the ribs); (2) create additional space for the upper part of the lungs by raising the shoulder girdle (collar bones, or clavicles); and/or (3) create space below the lungs by contracting the diaphragm.

In normal inhalation, only one-half liter of air is brought into the lungs; five times this amount can be inhaled by taking a deep breath. When we relax the muscles used in inhaling, one-half liter is again expelled without further muscle contraction. With deliberate exhalation through muscle contraction (abdominal muscles pushing diaphragm up and internal intercostal muscles reducing the circumference of the rib cage), additional liters of air are expelled. Thus we can speak of upper-chest breathing (clavicular breathing), lower-chest breathing, and diaphragmatic breathing. Females generally are supposed to employ more clavicular breathing, males more lower-chest breathing. (Few people other than singers employ diaphragmatic breathing except when lying down.) The explanation for the gender difference may be looked for in the fact that the breathing centers in the brain send out messages to all the muscles involved to start breathing; however, if certain muscles are placed under tension, either through posture (pulled-in stomach) or restrictive garments, the muscles may be hindered from taking part in the breathing process.

BREATHING EXERCISES

☐ In breathing exercises, we try to strengthen all the muscles involved in inhaling and exhaling. Some strengthening is accomplished through exercises not connected with breathing, such as sit-ups to firm the abdominal muscles or exercises to loosen the pectoral muscles so that the shoulders can be raised to expand the upper lobes of the lungs. However, there are special breathing exercises for the diaphragm and intercostal muscles which will help these muscles respond without effort to messages from the breathing center of the brain. Keep in mind that breathing not only clears carbon dioxide from the lungs and supplies oxygen to the hemoglobin molecules, but it also promotes the action of the skeletal muscle on which the lymphatic system depends for healthy functioning. The motion of the diaphragm is particularly important to promote drainage of lymph within the abdominal and thoracic cavities.

As with isometric exercise, it is best to isolate the various muscles to be trained for most efficient strengthening. We want to exercise separately, if possible, the muscles involved in clavicular, lower-chest, and diaphragmatic breathing. In order to do this, we first must become aware of these three types of breathing. This is not so easy, since when we breathe we usually don't pay attention to the fact that the way we are breathing changes automatically with our posture.

• An easy way to observe diaphragmatic breathing is to lie in bed in the fetal position and place one hand on the abdomen. You will observe how the hand moves out with the abdomen as you inhale, and how the hand moves in with the abdomen as you exhale. This is diaphragmatic breathing. As the diaphragm contracts, it creates more space for the lungs and at the same time it pushes the intestines down and the abdomen out. Relaxation of the diaphragm compresses the lungs; air is expelled and the abdomen retracts. By contracting the abdominal muscles deliberately, you push the diaphragm still farther up and expel more air. If you now turn on your back and keep your hand on your abdomen as you breathe (fig. 22), you are also able to purposefully increase the intensity of

**Breathing exercises,
figures 22–28**

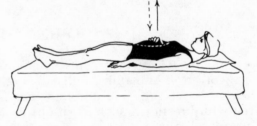

22. *Breathe by pushing
stomach out
(diaphragmatic
breathing).*

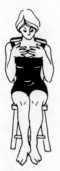

23. *Exhale, place hands
on upper chest,
fingertips touching.*

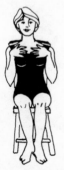

24. *Sit straight in chair
without leaning back,
inhale deeply
(clavicular breathing).
Notice fingertips move
apart slightly.*

breathing. This is easily done by breathing in and out through pursed lips (reducing the flow of air). You will immediately notice a stronger muscle action. If you breathe deeply in and out five times while observing the diaphragmatic action you will have done enough exercise for this part.

• Next, sit very straight on a chair without leaning against the back. Observe yourself in a mirror while you breathe. By sitting very straight you hold your stomach in, and this will prevent abdominal breathing. Now, lift your shoulders up and roll them slightly back. Breathe. You will observe your upper chest near the collar bone bulging a little as you inhale (figs. 23, 24). This is clavicular breathing. The collar bone and the shoulder blade are lifted to give the upper part of the rib cage and the tips of the lungs more freedom to expand. Breathe five times deeply through pursed lips; this trains the muscles needed for clavicular breathing.

• Next, still seated, lean back so that your shoulders touch the back of the chair. Place your fingers on the skin over the lower ribs and observe in the mirror how the fingertips move apart and come together again as the rib cage expands and contracts with inhaling and exhaling (figs. 25, 26). Breathe five times forcefully in and out through pursed lips. This exer-

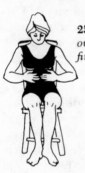

25. *Exhale, place hands
over lower ribs,
fingertips touching.*

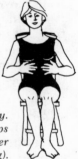

26. *Inhale deeply.
Notice fingertips
moving apart (lower
chest breathing).*

cises the intercostal muscles involved in lower-chest breathing. When you now place your hands on your abdomen, you probably will notice that when you breathe deeply, the diaphragm also is involved in pushing the stomach out (figs. 27, 28).

This upright position is ideal for relaxation and meditation. The gentle action of the diaphragm makes for highly efficient breathing, reducing the work of the heart. The blood tends to pool in the lower parts of the lungs, so oxygen is more readily exchanged for the waste gas, carbon dioxide.

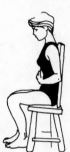

27. *Lean against back of chair, exhale.*

Once you have done breathing exercises a number of times, you will be able to observe that when you take a deep breath you utilize all three types of breathing: diaphragmatic, lower-chest, and clavicular. Note that in situations which trigger a nervous response, when the need for oxygen increases, you start to yawn, which involves all three types of breathing. Now you will have learned to utilize this very efficient type of breathing in all situations. It probably will be pleasant for you to take a few deep breaths during the day. Do not forget to exhale deliberately; exhaling (with contraction of muscles) is not part of our automatic breathing process, and doing it deliberately will help clear the lungs.

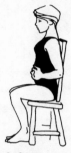

28. *Inhale. Notice stomach pushing out (diaphragmatic breathing).*

THE CIRCULATORY SYSTEM

□ The circulatory system works in close partnership with the respiratory system. As I have just described, the blood carries oxygen and nutrients to all the cells of the body, and picks up in exchange the waste products created in the process of burning energy. The lymphatic system, which I discuss in some detail in chapter 2, is also part of circulation and functions similarly to carry off wastes, most of which pass into the veins for eventual elimination.

Perhaps active people in normal good health need not think very much about these systems. But arthritics, because of their generally reduced level of activity, should be aware of them and should do what they can to keep them from getting sluggish, since this would mean a slowing down of the processes—so important for arthritics—of tissue rebuilding and especially of waste elimination.

EXERCISES FOR BETTER CIRCULATION

□ In this section, I give some circulation exercises that are suitable for most arthritics. Of course, the best exercise for circulation is brisk walking, and I hope you will make it part of your program so long as you are able to do so. But if you have chronic and severe arthritis, and can walk only with effort, there are alternative ways to exercise for better circulation. In my case, walking is out of the question; my limit without feeling fatigue is now fifty to one hundred slow paces. But I am able to do some efficient exercises for stimulating the heart rate to improve circulation. The exercises are suitable for almost everyone and can be used when brisk walking outdoors is impractical.

The first of these exercises is somewhat related to the strenuous push-ups that athletes do when in training, in which you lie prone and lift the upper body from the floor by straightening your arms (fig. 29). Exercising the upper extremities rapidly increases the blood pressure, which is why push-ups are so efficient for increasing circulation. The related exercise I recommend can be called the push-away.

Exercises for circulation, figures 29–32

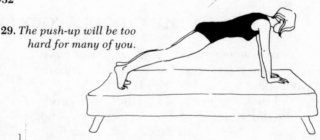

29. *The push-up will be too hard for many of you.*

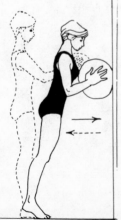

• Stand a few feet away from the wall. Let yourself fall forward toward the wall and push away again with your hands.

Here is a variation for those with arthritis in the wrists, for whom pushing away with the hands would cause discomfort. Hold a beach ball in front of you as you fall toward the wall (fig. 30). Push away the beach ball to bring yourself back to the upright position.

30. *Push yourself off the wall until you are tired. Use a ball to protect your hands.*

Repeat this exercise, with or without the ball, until your heart rate increases (to be discussed with your physician) or until you feel you have had a sufficient workout. The push-aways from the wall have the same effect as push-ups in stimulating circulation, although you must do more of them to achieve a similar rise in heart rate.

The second exercise is related to knee-bends. Time was when I could do twenty to thirty knee-bends at my physician's request, so that he could check on how long it took for my increased pulse rate to return to normal. Now, I find this too strenuous, although it is an excellent workout for the lower extremities. Here is an easier version that will be suitable for almost everyone, except perhaps those who are having problems with their hips.

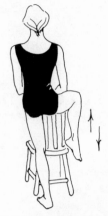

31 & 32. *Walk in place as fast as you like. Lean your hands on the back of a chair.*

• Stand in back of a chair, bending over slightly and supporting yourself on the back of the chair (fig. 31). Raise one leg with the knee bent and bring it down, then raise the other leg with the knee bent and bring it down (fig. 32). Repeat this sequence, at first slowly and then, perhaps, a little more quickly as you get the feel of it. Continue until you feel your heart rate going up, or until you feel you have had an adequate workout. Attaching an ankle weight will speed the process. It will take considerably longer to increase your heart rate by means of raising your legs than by pushing yourself away from the wall, and the blood pressure is not as easily increased by means of exercising the lower extremities as it is by exercising the upper ones.

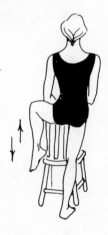

HOW TO INVENT YOUR OWN EXERCISES

☐ The two exercises I have described are meant for increasing general circulation and for increasing the heart rate. It makes sense to do them in the same exercise session so that you push blood into both the lower and upper extremities. Some may not care for or may not be able to do either of these exercises. (For example, since I developed more difficulty with one hip, I cannot carry out the leg-raising exercise without pain.) If the movements are too difficult or cause pain, try thinking up exercises of your own. For instance, you can lie down and move your legs by extending them and flexing them. Strenuous exertion is not essential to these exercises; it's the repetition that increases the heart rate.

LOCALIZED CIRCULATION

□ Apart from the stimulation of the heart rate for allover circulation, there is considerable importance attached to localized circulation, the flow of blood and lymph in isolated parts of the body. We have all had the experience at one time or another of having a foot "fall asleep" because we were inactive or kept a leg in a cramped position for too long. What I do in such instances is to sit in a chair with my foot on the floor and raise the heel so that the foot is supported just by the toes. By rapidly contracting and relaxing the calf muscle, I can shake the whole leg up and down. In less than a half-minute, the circulation is back to normal and the tingling feeling has vanished. There you have a method for exercising almost any part of the body to speed up circulation, whether it is the arm or leg, wrist or ankle. Merely move the arm or leg rhythmically back and forth to restore circulation. This type of exercise is useful, too, when a joint becomes chilled.

Have you ever gotten very cold and begun to shiver? The shivering is the body's defense reaction to cold. It activates the muscles and quickly generates heat in the body. When you shake a part of the body to restore circulation you are imitating the body's normal response to the cold.

CHILLED JOINTS

□ A simpler way, certainly, is to prevent cold from affecting your joints. This can be damaging, since a chilled joint may be strained if it is suddenly put to use. If my ankles become very cold, that means circulation in them is sluggish, and if I then get up and start to walk briskly or perform some other rapid activity involving the ankles, I am likely to provoke pain, indicating that some slight damage or stress has occurred. If you disregard such pains, they are liable to set in and remain for a long time, requiring heat treatments and the like. Therefore, I advise that you be sure your joints are warm before you use them; particularly in cold weather, make use of woollen warmers for the wrists, knees, shoulders, ankles, wherever you need them (See Directory of Aids. See also figure 42, page 270). Women in winter are particularly vulnerable to chilled ankles.

If you live in a cold climate, I am sure you are accustomed to wearing a scarf during the winter to protect your neck. What happens if you don't protect your neck? You may get a chill followed by muscle spasms —the so-called stiff neck. This can happen to anyone, arthritic or not, so we learn to prevent it by wearing a scarf. Now with arthritis, the whole body needs the same kind of protection. We have to tread on the careful side and protect our joints. We have to wear our scarfs, knee warmers, and so forth, and if these are not enough to fend off the cold, then we have to increase our localized circulation by means of exercise.

10

Friday Night: Hips, Lower Back, and Knees

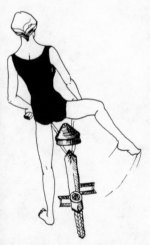

1 & 2. *Becoming aware of hip motion*

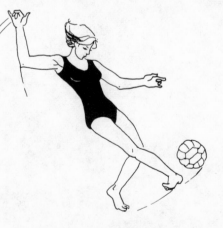

□ The hips (which move the legs) are not quite as mobile as the shoulders (which move the arms), but they have far more mobility than we aware of (figs. 1, 2). The game of soccer offers a remarkable demonstration of hip mobility. In soccer, a player's hip has to be flexed or extended in various positions as the upper leg is rotated and the foot brought in contact with the ball at all possible angles. The hip also absorbs the forces transmitted from impact with the ball.

Rheumatologists call the hip a weight-bearing joint, meaning that it is one of the joints that support the weight of the body. If you stand on one foot, your body weight, minus the weight of the leg you are standing on, will be resting on your hip joint. Actually, the forces acting on the hip in a perpendicular direction are greater than the body weight. This has to do with kinetic energy. For example, when you jump onto one leg, even if it is just a small jump of, say, an inch or two, this transmits an impact to the joints. When you walk slowly, you transmit little more than a static force to the hip joints with each step. However, as you walk more briskly, or start to jog or run, the velocity of the motion is such that a force greater than the static weight of the body is exerted on the hip joint, though for a shorter period of time. The principle of impact is demonstrated when you hammer a nail into a piece of wood. If you merely rest the hammer on top of the nail, the nail will not enter the wood. But if you let the hammer drop from the height of one or two inches, the impact will drive it somewhat into the wood. If you exert some swinging force onto the hammer, the nail will be driven easily into the wood. The impact, called kinetic force, is proportional to the square of the velocity of the hammer coming down onto the nail. Applying this principle to the force that is transmitted to the hip from a foot touching the ground in human motion, we see that when we walk twice as fast, four times the force is loaded onto the hip, even though for a shorter period of time. When we run, moving at about four times our normal speed, the hip absorbs sixteen times the amount of static force, again for a shorter period of time. From this analysis we can readily understand the need for strengthening the muscles around the weight-bearing joints. These muscles have to stabilize a force of several times the weight of the body, that is, several hundred pounds. During isometric exercise, we try to simulate these forces by tensing our muscles in opposition to immobile objects.

THE BENEFITS OF BRISK WALKING

☐ A muscle that is maintained at its fullest normal length is more efficient, and therefore stronger, than a muscle that has been allowed to shorten slightly. Constant use of muscles tends to shorten them, so it is important to maintain their length through exercise.

The best exercise for the muscles of the weight-bearing joints is to walk briskly. A slow walk will not exercise the muscle through its full range, nor will it exert maximum force on the muscles. Walking briskly for a short period of time is more efficient in building strength than walking slowly for a longer period of time. Unfortunately, we arthritics tend to walk very slowly, and all the more slowly the longer we have arthritis. Our joints are sensitive and we shy away from the normal impacts of brisk walking and running. As a consequence, our muscles become weaker and the vicious cycle of inactivity is reinforced.

THE HIP JOINT

☐ At the hip joint, the spherical end of the femur fits snugly into the part of the pelvis called the acetabulum (fig. 3). (Acetabulum, from the Latin, means "vessel containing vinegar"; evidently the bony formation is similar in shape to the vinegar cruet used on Roman tables.) Whereas, in the shoulder, the various directions of motion are governed by a number of joints belonging to the shoulder complex, at either side of the hip a single joint controls all motions while also bearing the weight of the body. This results in considerable stress and wear on the hip joint, to the point where it may eventually become unstable, produc-

3. *Hip joint and total hip replacement*

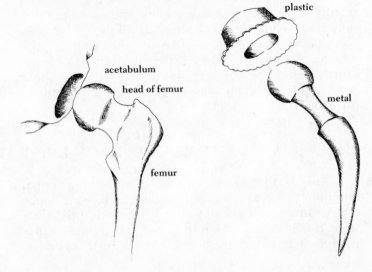

acetabulum

head of femur

femur

plastic

metal

ing disability and pain. Daily range-of-motion and strengthening exercises are very important at the onset of instability so that some degree of functioning and comfort can be maintained. Such exercises have helped me considerably. Nowadays arthritics have the option of total hip replacement (fig. 3), a surgical procedure that is carried out widely with a high degree of success. However, since there are always some risks involved, such operations are usually delayed until the discomfort and disability of the hip problem have become insupportable. So long as the condition is bearable, the arthritic's best choice is to stay as comfortable as possible, use the least encumbering assistive appliance (such as one or two canes or a forearm crutch), and exercise to maintain the greatest possible degree of mobility.

TESTING THE HIP RANGES

□ In the pages that follow, I will describe movements to test the ranges of the hip, then range-of-motion exercises, then stretching exercises for the muscles involved in locomotion, and finally strengthening exercises for those muscles. With hip muscles that are weak after prolonged bed rest, it may be best to reverse the sequence: to do isometric strengthening first, then gradually introduce range-of-motion exercises. This, I have found, can be the least painful and most efficient way to make progress.

• To test the hip, lie down with two pillows supporting the upper back so that you can observe well what you are doing (fig. 4). With the left leg stretched out, bend the right knee, place the right heel on your left thigh, slightly above your left knee, and move your right thigh and knee slowly down toward the surface of the bed as far as you can. There should be no pain; if there is, report it to your physician or therapist.

Complementary Exercise

Repeat the same exercise for the other hip by touching the left foot to the thigh above the right knee and letting the left knee sink to the surface of the bed (fig. 5). This will test the hip for *f*lexion, *ab*duction, and *ex*ternal *r*otation (*faber*).

**Testing the hip ranges,
figures 4–13**

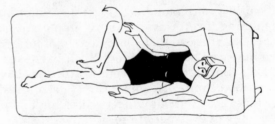

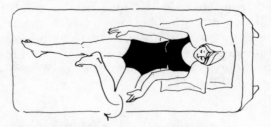

4 & 5. *This tests for flexion, abduction and external rotation (faber).*

If you have become accustomed to crossing your legs in this way while you sit on a chair (fig. 6), you also will have checked and exercised the above-mentioned ranges of the hip. The Yoga lotus position also exercises the faber ranges. *Do not attempt it* if you have arthritis, as it places an excessive strain on ligaments (fig. 7).

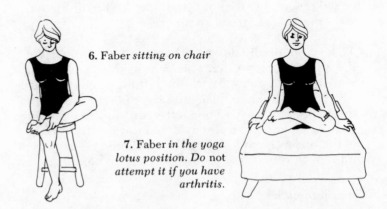

6. Faber *sitting on chair*

7. Faber *in the yoga lotus position. Do not attempt it if you have arthritis.*

• To test internal rotation of the hip, lie on your back on the bed. Flex the knees, then move the right knee closer to the ground by gliding the right heel to the right on the surface of the bed (fig. 8).

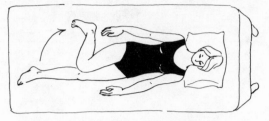

8 & 9. *This tests flexion, adduction and internal rotation.*

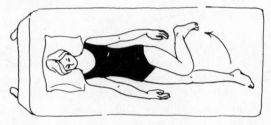

Complementary Exercise

Repeat this for the other leg (fig. 9).

- To test the extension of the left hip (fig. 10), bring your right knee close to your chest while lying down and try to keep your left leg flat on the ground. If the flexor is tight, the left knee will automatically rise a little. The hip is extended when you lie on your stomach (fig. 11a).

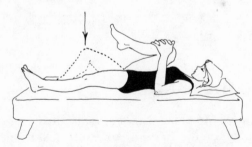

10 & 11. *Try to keep straight leg flat on the bed. This tests for hip flexion (one leg), extension (other leg).*

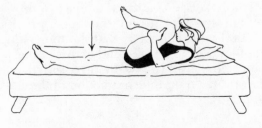

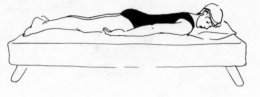

11a. *Lying on your stomach for half an hour each day prevents flexion contraction.*

Complementary Exercise

Repeat the test for the other leg (fig. 11).

12 & 13. *Abduction and external rotation of the hips*

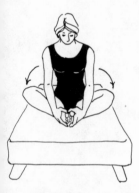

12. *With hips flexed*

• To test external rotation and abduction, sit upright on the bed with your knees spread apart and try to touch your feet with your hands (fig. 12).
• External and internal rotation are also tested with the leg straight. Keep legs slightly apart while lying down with your **upper back** supported so that you can observe your legs. Roll legs in and then out. Observe knees and feet, which should show a rotation of about forty-five degrees (fig. 13).

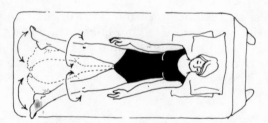

13. *With hips extended*

EXERCISING THE HIP RANGES

☐ We move now from movements designed to test your range of hip motion to exercises designed to maintain and extend those ranges.

• External and internal rotation with the knees and legs straight: Exercise these ranges in the same position you used for testing them (see previous exercise). Roll your legs in so that the toes point toward each other (fig. 13). At the end of this range, tense the leg muscles as if you wanted to roll the legs still farther in. Hold up the contraction of the muscles for about three seconds (count of six). Relax. Then roll feet outward so that feet and knees are pointed out (fig. 13). Strain your muscles at the end of this range, as if you wanted to turn the legs farther out. Hold the contraction for three seconds (count of six). Relax. Now, roll feet inward again. Complete tense-relax procedure as outlined above a few times for both the internal and external rotation. You will notice that you either gradually increase the rotation or, at least, that you reach the end of the range with less tension, which means that you have succeeded in loosening the muscles somewhat.

• In this exercise, you try to overcome the tension of the very powerful adductor muscles, which bring legs together.

Lie down with your upper back supported so that you can observe the exercise position. Spread your legs as widely apart as possible (fig. 14). Strain your leg muscles as if you wanted to bring the legs together but were prevented from doing so by some resisting force. (Until you become aware of these muscles, your therapist or helper can provide you with resistance on the inside of the legs, against which you strain.) Tense for three seconds (count of six). Relax. Try to move legs farther apart. Repeat this procedure a few times. You will notice that it gradually becomes easier to spread the legs apart, and gain a little range.

One way I supply resistance for the adductors is to dig my heels strongly into the bed and strain the adductor muscles as if to bring my legs together. In doing this, keep the legs straight.

Another way is to slide the foot just beyond the edge of the bed and press the foot against the edge of the bed, to the count of six, keeping the leg straight. Relax, then once you are able to spread your legs so that both feet are beyond the edges of the bed, press

Tense-relax, and stretch your muscles for all positions shown, figures 14–25

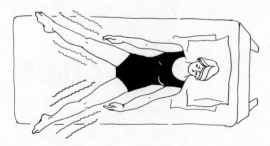

14. *Tighten the leg muscles, relax, then spread legs.*

with both feet against the bed to the count of six, keeping the legs straight. Relax, and move legs farther out. I have found my twin size bed (thirty-nine inches or one meter wide) just the right size for this purpose.

In the next three exercises, abduction as well as internal and external rotation of the thigh are exercised with the hip in flexed position, that is, with the leg at a ninety-degree angle to the trunk. The knees are usually kept flexed for these exercises, because the straight leg at ninety degrees to the trunk introduces additional tension, namely that of the hamstring muscles. We want to avoid, if possible, dealing with a multitude of tense muscles at the same time, since we want to concentrate our awareness on the muscle we are working with.

• Lying flat on your back on the bed (you may want to place a small pillow under the head), lift your right knee so that the thigh is about ninety degrees to the bed (fig. 15). The knee may be flexed for comfort. Now, abduct the right leg by spreading it outward as far as it will go (fig. 16). Contract your adductor muscles by straining those muscles which would bring the leg back to the starting position, but do not actually perform the movement. You can touch the adductor muscles on the inside of your thigh to observe how they contract. Hold the contraction for about

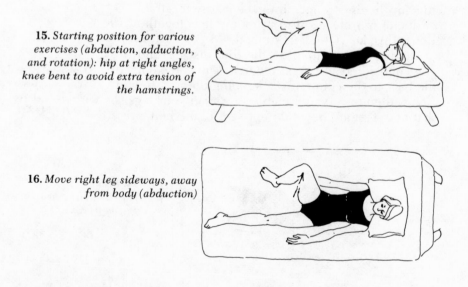

15. *Starting position for various exercises (abduction, adduction, and rotation): hip at right angles, knee bent to avoid extra tension of the hamstrings.*

16. *Move right leg sideways, away from body (abduction)* three seconds (count of six). Relax, then try to abduct the leg a little farther. Repeat a few times if you feel that there is some stiffness to overcome.

- Move the leg back to the starting position (fig. 15), with the thigh at right angles to the bed. Now, rotate your right leg in such a way that your right foot swings toward the left as far as possible while the knee remains in place (fig. 17). This accomplishes external rotation of the thigh; the normal range is forty-five degrees.

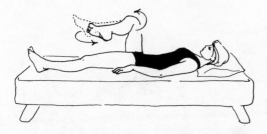

17. *Swing right foot to left to rotate hip externally. Assume the thigh to be a crank and the foot to be its handle. As you swing the handle the crank will rotate in one or the other direction.*

If you feel stiffness or want to increase your range, contract your muscles as if you wanted to move your foot away from the center line of the body, but without actually doing so. Some resistance to the foot is useful and this can be supplied with your left knee. Keep up the contraction for two to three seconds (count of six). Relax, then try to rotate the leg a little farther.

- Next, go back to the starting position shown in figure 15. Now rotate the right thigh inward by swinging the foot outward as far as possible (fig. 18). The normal range, again, is 45 degrees. If improvement is needed, tense your muscles as if to bring the foot back toward the center line of the body but without actually moving it. Hold the contraction for three seconds (count of six). Relax, and try to swing the foot farther out so that the thigh rotates farther inward.

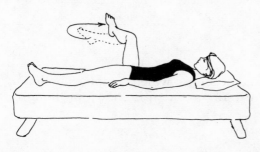

18. *Swing the foot outward to rotate the thigh (crank inward).*

Complementary Exercises

Repeat the three preceding exercises with the *left* leg.
From the starting position (fig. 15), with the right leg
straight on the bed, raise the left knee so that the thigh
is at right angles to the bed. Abduct the left leg by
moving it down toward the bed (fig. 19). Externally
rotate the left thigh by rotating the foot inward (fig.
20). Internally rotate the left thigh by rotating the foot
outward (fig. 21). Tense the muscles at the ends of the
ranges for about three seconds (count of six). Relax,
and try to extend the ranges.

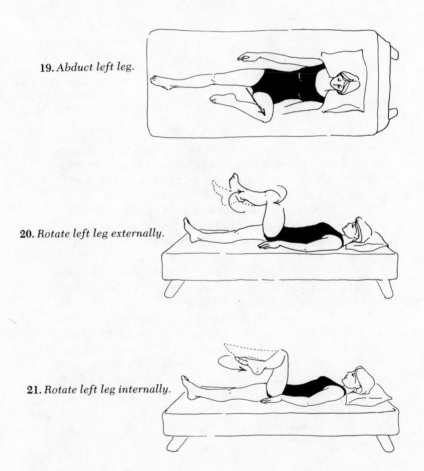

19. *Abduct left leg.*

20. *Rotate left leg externally.*

21. *Rotate left leg internally.*

A very important exercise which combines both hip
abduction and external rotation is shown in the next
three figures.

• Lie on the bed with your legs straight and together, and the upper back supported so that you can see what you are doing. Next, move both heels, on the surface of the bed, toward your buttocks, with knees abducted as far as possible from the center line of the body (fig. 22). Try to sit up and grasp your feet. If not possible, grasp the lower legs and try to pull the legs toward the chest, keeping the knees abducted as far as possible (fig. 23). Try to increase the ranges; that is, try to bring the feet closer to the buttocks and to further abduct the knees. You can aid this by first tensing the adductor muscles, which act to bring the legs together. These are the antagonist muscles that move the legs in the opposite direction of the exercise motion of abduction. After you have strongly tensed and then relaxed these muscles, they give less resistance to the abductor muscles and the external rotators, so that the legs move farther in the desired direction. Tense for three seconds at a time (count of six), then relax for a second or so. Move heels closer to the body and the knees lower to the bed. In this position the legs form a diamond shape. This exercise, much favored by ballet dancers, is extremely efficient in maintaining flexibility of the hip.

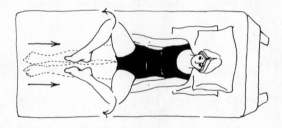

22. Produce a diamond shape with your legs.

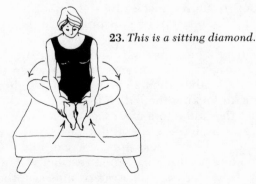

23. This is a sitting diamond.

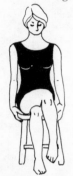

24. *Once more; this is the preferred way of sitting with crossed legs.*

25. *This position is inadvisable if it produces pain.*

In daily life, if you want to cross your legs, you should do it as shown in figure 24. The ankle is resting on the thigh or knee of the other leg; the knee is abducted as much as possible. Become accustomed to doing this sometimes with one leg and sometimes with the other. In this way you will exercise both of your hips. You may lean gently down onto the abducted knee to extend your range, but do not lean heavily so as to produce pain. (A good time and place to practice this, I found, is when you are sitting on a step in a thermal pool. With my muscles relaxed by the warm water, I was able to bring the knee further down by pumping it gently five or ten times. Never try, however, to reach beyond the limit of pain.)

The other way of sitting with crossed legs, with one thigh over the other and the lower legs parallel (fig. 25), is not a good position if it produces pain. Although the hip abductors are stretched in this position, the whole hip joint is subjected to abnormal stress. After one of my hip joints had become unstable, crossing my legs in this way became quite painful. In daily life, this adducted position of the leg is rarely used, and I don't see much sense in practicing it with exercises. However, this does not contradict the advice about the need to maintain the strength of adductor muscles through isometric exercise; they are essential for the stability of the hip joints, as will be described later.

THE MUSCLES OF THE LEG

☐ Let us take some time to get better acquainted with the various muscles that move the lower extremities. In this section I give you some special stretching exercises for these muscles (figs. 26, 27).

I have already told you how to feel the adductor muscles on the inside of the thighs as you bring your legs together against resistance. These are quite powerful muscles, and one may wonder when they come into play, other than in holding onto a horse while riding, or kicking the ball sideways in soccer. The fact is that the adductors are essential for the stability of the legs. So too are the abductor muscles, which are located in the buttocks area; you can feel them twitch as you abduct the leg against resistance. On the front of the thighs are the quadriceps muscles; they extend the knees, and one section helps to flex the hips. On the back of the thighs are the hamstrings.

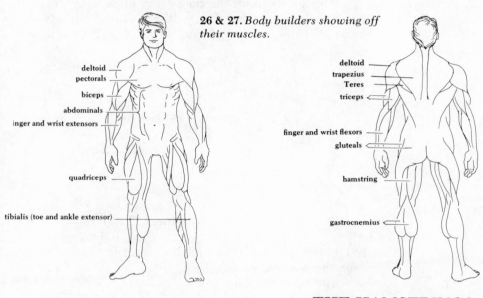

26 & 27. *Body builders showing off their muscles.*

deltoid
pectorals
biceps
abdominals
finger and wrist extensors
quadriceps
tibialis (toe and ankle extensor)

deltoid
trapezius
Teres
triceps
finger and wrist flexors
gluteals
hamstring
gastrocnemius

THE HAMSTRINGS

☐ The hamstring is a very powerful muscle which flexes the knee and extends the hip. In order to stretch this muscle, you have to move in the direction opposite to its action; that is, flex the hip and extend the knee. There are various ways to do this necessary stretching. When we were young, we used to stretch this muscle by bending over with knees straight and trying to touch the floor (fig. 28). Do not attempt this if you have severe arthritis, unless you can reach your toes easily without any undue tension. My rheumatologist warned me that exerting too much effort in trying to touch the floor was potentially harmful for the back, and I repeat his warning here.

Stretching of the hamstring muscle, figures 28–32

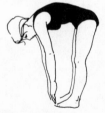

28. *Touching toes is considered too strenuous for the arthritic.*

• For arthritics, a better way to stretch the hamstrings is to lie down and lift one leg straight up to at least a right angle (fig. 29). To extend the range, it is usually

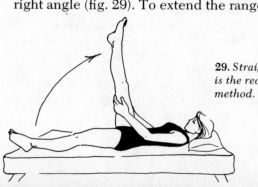

29. *Straight leg raises is the recommended method.*

recommended to lift the leg many times; the typical prescription is to raise each leg ten times.

I prefer to warm up the hamstring muscle by digging the heel into the bed with the knee slightly flexed for three seconds (count of six) (fig. 29a), and

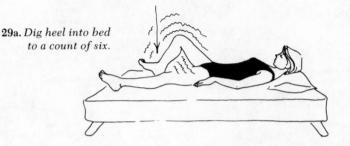

29a. *Dig heel into bed to a count of six.*

then lifting the leg again. It is ideal if a therapist or helper provides resistance and then moves your straight leg passively as high as possible until you reach the point of pain. When exercising alone, I am also able to extend my leg farther by grasping the straight leg with both hands and moving it up (fig. 30). For this purpose it is best not to lie completely flat; use pillows to raise your upper torso.

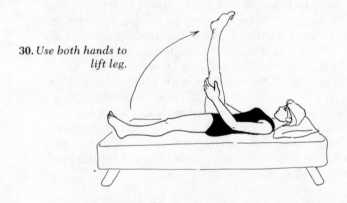

30. *Use both hands to lift leg.*

In stretching the hamstring, more than with any other muscle, I can feel the stretching in the area of the muscle itself, rather than in the neighboring joints. When I do the hamstring stretch with my therapist, she usually watches my face and at the first sign of pain, we stop the stretch. I have observed how athletes massage their hamstring muscles while stretching them, and I have tried the same thing with success. It may be difficult for you to reach the back of your thigh to massage the hamstring and you may not have enough strength in your hands to provide a deep kneading action. I have found that just stroking the muscle and stretching the skin with my fingers provides a kind of counterirritant action which seems to make the discomfort from stretching more acceptable and permit the stretching to be carried a little bit farther.

The hamstring muscle seems to tighten up easily. I find its range quite reduced every time I resume stretching after a period of inactivity, and it is gratifying to see how much the range improves with exercise. The hamstring muscle seems to require many repetitions of the stretching exercise, even after it has been warmed up. I encourage you to persevere in this important stretching, since a shortened hamstring can contribute not only to hip instability, but to lower back trouble as well.

• You can also stretch the hamstring muscle while sitting on a bed with your legs outstretched and reaching with the arms toward the toes (fig. 31). Between stretches, tense the muscle by digging in the heels with the knees slightly bent.

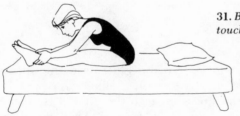

31. *Bend forward to touch your toes.*

32. *Or on two chairs.*

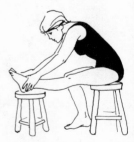

You can also sit on the edge of the bed or on a chair and place your feet on the seat of a chair of the same or slightly lower height. Figure 32 shows one leg supported on the chair and the other one on the floor. This permits stretching the hamstring muscle of one leg at a time, just as in leg-raising. I find this position more comfortable for my unstable hip than lying down and raising the leg. Avoid abrupt and jerky movements in leg-raising exercises, otherwise the hip joint can be put under pressure, producing pain.

THE GLUTEALS (BUTTOCKS)

Stretching of the buttock muscles (gluteals), figures 33–35

☐ Next, we come to stretching the gluteals, or buttock muscles, which come into play when we extend the leg or abduct it. A common exercise for stretching the gluteals is to bring one thigh, then the other thigh (fig. 33), and finally both thighs (fig. 34) close to the chest while you are lying down. You may support your upper torso while doing this in order to be more comfortable.

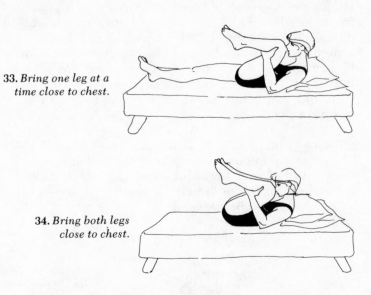

33. *Bring one leg at a time close to chest.*

34. *Bring both legs close to chest.*

35. *Omit if this puts too much strain on your spine.*

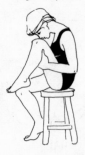

• I prefer to stretch the gluteals while sitting on the edge of the bed or on a chair. Grasping the thigh, bring the knee close to the chest (try to touch your nose with your knee, fig. 35). This stretches the gluteals and also provides a slight stretch to the lower back region. It helps if you pull your stomach in while you do this exercise.

After I bring each knee close to my nose, I abduct the knee slowly as far as it will go (moving it to one side), then I adduct the knee slowly, returning it toward the center line of the body.

The warm-up of the gluteals between stretches can be done by pressing the thigh against both forearms for three seconds (count of six), relaxing, then pulling the thigh with the forearms toward your chest and nose.

THE HIP FLEXORS

☐ The next muscles to be stretched are the hip flexors. Stretching the hip flexors, as well as the gluteals and the hamstrings, helps keep the lower back limber.

• Lie on your stomach and raise your legs as high as possible, one at a time (fig. 36). The second part of this exercise requires a therapist or helper who will support your thigh and provide resistance for your hip flexors to warm them up and stabilize your pelvis. Press the thigh against the resisting hands for three seconds (count of six), then relax and permit the leg to be lifted higher.

Stretching the hip flexors, or extension of the hip, figures 36 & 37

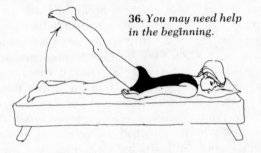

36. *You may need help in the beginning.*

• Another way to stretch the hip flexors is to lie on your back and bring one knee at a time as close to the chest as possible while lowering the other leg, held straight, slowly to the bed (fig. 37). At the end of the range you will notice a considerable tension which will force you to sit up a little higher. Raising the straight leg a few inches and holding it there for a few seconds exercises the hip flexors efficiently to warm them up and may permit a slightly increased stretch.

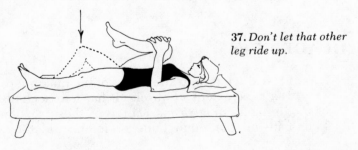

37. *Don't let that other leg ride up.*

CAUTIONS FOR THOSE WITH
LOWER BACK TROUBLE

☐ People with lower back trouble should consult a physician or therapist promptly if any pain at all is felt while doing these exercises. In some cases a program for strengthening the abdominal muscles and the lower back muscles may have to be carried out before the person can start stretching the muscles mentioned above. Any pain in the buttock area or in the legs, even without pain in the lower back, may indicate a sciatica condition which will require extended periods of rest in a comfortable, pain-free position. An example is the fetal position (fig. 38), in which you lie on your side with legs pulled in and back curved. I had such a condition at one time and could not lie for long on my side before my hip started to hurt. A pillow between the knees or thighs helped this somewhat. The pain of sciatica may be due to compression of a nerve root by an intervertebral disk. I was most comfortable while in bed when I had the upper torso supported by two or three pillows and one or two pillows raising the knees. This position relaxes most of those leg muscles which can produce tightness around the lower back and thereby increase pain. At the same time, it causes the lower back to be slightly curved, thereby relieving pressure on the intervertebral disks.

Such lower back conditions usually quiet down with rest. Exercises for the lower back help to keep this area and the pelvis limber and strong and thus they help prevent recurrence of the back trouble.

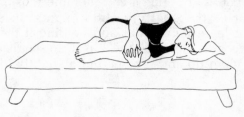

38. *Fetal position, specially comfortable in case of lower back trouble.*

THE QUADRICEPS

☐ Next we turn to stretching of the quadriceps, which is a knee extensor muscle. It has four sections, hence the name *quadriceps*. Three of these sections originate on the thigh bone or femur and they can be stretched by flexing the knee as much as possible while the hip also is flexed.

• You may do this either while sitting or while lying on your side or back, in bed or in a warm bath (fig. 39). Bend your knee passively by holding the leg around the shin bone and bringing the knee close to your chest.

Stretching the quadriceps, figures 39–42

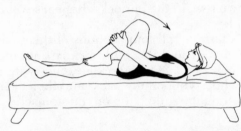

39. *Hand around the shinbone, pull toward chest. Stop short of pain in the knee.*

Warming up this muscle to increase the range can be accomplished by extending the knee against hand pressure on the shin bone for three seconds (count of six); relax and stretch some more. Stop short of pain in your knee. Repeat until there is no more improvement during the session.

Complementary Exercise

Repeat exercise with the other leg.

• You can also exercise the quadriceps muscles prior to stretching them by using ankle weights (fig. 40). Lying on your back, with knees toward chest, lift a weighted ankle (start with two-pound weights) a few inches, then relax quadriceps muscles, letting the heel fall toward the buttocks. Repeat this procedure several times with each leg. Pain in the knee is a limiting factor. Respect it.

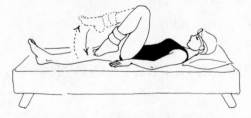

40. *Let the ankle weight pull your foot toward the buttocks. Swing foot up and let it drop down.*

One quadriceps muscle section originates in the pelvis and acts in flexing the hip as well as extending the knee.

• To stretch this section, lie on your stomach and flex the knee as much as possible with a slow whipping motion (fig. 41). Stop if you feel pain. To warm up this muscle before stretching it, use resistance provided by your helper or else use ankle weights. Lie on the bed on your stomach with the knees flexed, and try to lift the ankle weight for a count of two or three. Relax the quadriceps muscles and let the leg drop down toward the buttocks. Repeat several times for both legs.

In this fashion, all four sections of the quadriceps are stretched. I find it useful to carry out both types of stretches; that is, I flex the knee, once with the hip flexed (while lying on my back) and then again with the hip straight (while lying on my stomach).

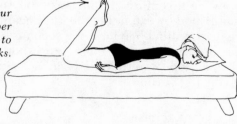

41. *You may tense your quadriceps in the upper thigh, relax, then try to whip feet toward buttocks.*

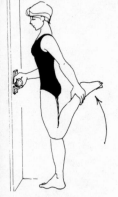

42. *Do this one only if you are steady on one leg.*

Here, finally, is another efficient stretch for the quadriceps which you do while standing. I don't recommend it unless you are quite stable on your legs.

• Stand on one leg and support yourself by holding on to the back of a chair. Bend the free leg and grasp it at the ankle (fig. 42). Pull the heel toward the buttock as far as possible.

Complementary Exercise

Repeat exercise with the other leg.

PENDULUM MOVEMENTS FOR PASSIVE STRETCHING

☐ Here are two more stretching exercises, which I will call knee-swinging and hip-swinging. They are similar to the pendulum exercise described for the shoulder in chapter 7.

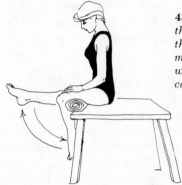

43. *Swing one knee up, the other one down all the way. Repeat as many times as you wish, to loosen knee capsule.*

Pendulum exercises for the hip, figures 44 & 45

• For the knees, sit on a sturdy table with your lower legs dangling; you can put a rolled-up towel under your thighs for comfort. Now swing your lower leg forward and back (fig. 43). Swing first one leg and then the other, or both together. Do up to twenty swings, forward and back. Exert as little muscular force as possible; use momentum to accomplish the swinging motion. You should try, however, to bring the legs up so that the knee is straight when swinging forward, and this may require some tensing of the quadriceps. After sufficient practice, you will be swinging the legs forward with momentum and will not need to tense the quadriceps.

The idea of this exercise is to keep the knee capsule loose. I had a long-standing condition of pain from a tendon that moved across the bony prominence of the knee joint when I bent or extended my knee. The problem subsided after three weeks of daily swinging exercises.

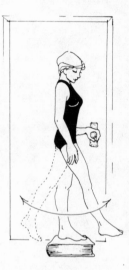

44. *Swing hip slowly back and forth. Feel the weight of the leg. Be sure to hold on tightly to doorknob or chair back.*

• To do the swinging exercise for the hip, stand with one foot on a thick book or similar platform holding onto a door handle or the back of a chair for stability (fig. 44). Let the free leg hang limply down, then swing it gently forward and backward. Get a feel for the weight of your leg and imagine that your leg is a pendulum with the weight concentrated in the foot. As you start to swing the leg very gently forward and backward, try not to tense any muscles. Do this slowly up to ten to twenty times for each leg.

A variation of this exercise, leg-circling, is also very beneficial. Support yourself by holding onto a doorknob or chair back. Stand on one foot and de-

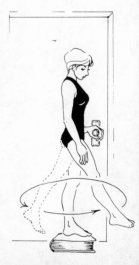

45. *Letting leg hang down limply, try to describe circles with your foot.*

scribe the largest possible circle with the other leg
—forward, sideways, and backward. Do this a few
times for each leg (fig. 45).

STRENGTHENING THE LOWER BACK

☐ We now turn to muscle strengthening. I will first
describe muscle strengthening for the lower back,
which goes hand in hand with stretching of the gluteals and hamstring muscles.

Normally, the lumbar portion of the spine is slightly
curved (fig. 46). The five lumbar vertebrae (called L_1,
L_2, . . . L_5) are large vertebrae which, together with the
intervertebral disks and the first sacral vertebra (S_1),
which is firmly connected to the pelvis, behave in a
manner similar to a joint. That is, they permit the
upper spine to flex and extend, and to rotate and swing
sideways. If you sit squarely on a stool and bend your
torso in various directions, it is accomplished through
the flexibility of the lumbar spine. The biggest stress
is absorbed by the disk between L_5 and S_1. If the muscles that stabilize the position of the vertebrae are
weak, a jerky motion may make the disk protrude,
thereby impinging on nerve roots that lie very close
by. This may produce irritation and even damage to
the powerful sciatic nerve, with resulting severe pain
and even numbness along the buttocks and legs. In
most cases, we are told, this condition repairs itself if
we rest in a comfortable position, such as the fetal
position (fig. 38). Once the pain has subsided, exercises are started.

46. *The lumbar spine is*
flexible and borders on the
sacral vertebrae, which are
connected to the pelvis.

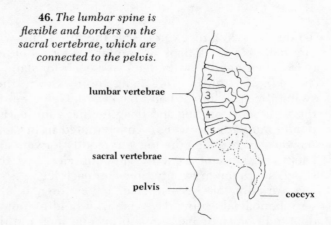

lumbar vertebrae

sacral vertebrae

pelvis

coccyx

Once, when I was away on vacation I had a severe
attack of sciatica. Not wanting to spend the time in
bed—indeed, having a hard time finding any comfortable position at all—I decided to try acupuncture
treatment, which I received from a Chinese physician
in Palm Springs, California. The treatments proved
highly effective. The doctor inserted a needle in the
L_5-S_1 region, and further needles in a particularly
painful area in my buttocks and in the lower leg, sup-
posedly in the path of the sciatic nerve. All the
needles were interconnected by wires leading to a box
that supplied pulsating current, which the doctor adjusted to tolerance. Each treatment lasted twenty to
thirty minutes. After three daily treatments, the pain
was sufficiently reduced so I could sleep at night without being propped up by a variety of pillows under the
knees and upper back. The doctor suggested daily
treatments on other parts of the body, to which I con-
sented, more out of curiosity than any conviction that
they would do anything further for my sciatica. I was
rewarded by having a pain of long standing removed
in a carpal-metacarpal joint of my left thumb. This permitted me to exercise this thumb vigorously and improve the grip of my left hand.

After I communicated the favorable result of my
acupuncture treatments to some of my fellow vacation-
ers, they introduced me to a lady who had undergone
disk surgery, which left some unaccounted-for severe
pains. She had obtained an initial acupuncture treatment and later underwent TNS—transcutaneous
nerve stimulation—at the pain clinic of the University
of California Medical School in Los Angeles. This
three-month course of treatment apparently eliminated the pain; it had not recurred in the half-year
since she stopped treatment, and she was pursuing
normal activities.

In TNS, small electrodes are applied to the surface
of the skin, at the same points that are chosen for the
insertion of the acupuncture needles. The electrodes
are wired to a pulsating electricity generator similar to
the one used in my acupuncture treatments. Although
I have not undergone TNS, it is evident to me that
both this technique and acupuncture can eliminate
certain types of pain, in many cases. Sciatica seems to
be amenable to these procedures. However, these procedures are not curative. In my case, as was predict-
able, the body repaired itself after having had enough

rest; the acupuncture helped me to be more comfortable during this period. After this body self-repair, however, I was aware of the need to strengthen and stretch the appropriate muscles so as to prevent undue tension on the lower back and stabilize it to prevent recurrence of the back trouble.

I think it is useful to tell you some of my own experiences with back trouble, as well as the modalities and types of exercise which seemed to help me. Evidently the potential for low back problems is great, and I would like to stress prevention. I describe muscle strengthening for the abdominal muscles as well as the lower back muscles and gluteals as part of the weekly routine. The stretching of gluteals, hamstrings, and the hip flexors, often prescribed for lower back problems, is part of exercises for the hips.

If you have lower back problems, please do not rely on this chapter as the only source of guidance on what to do. There are a number of good books that go into the subject more extensively. Most important, you should consult your physician for proper diagnosis if pain persists and your back doesn't seem to repair itself after you have rested for some time. Your physician will want to have X-rays made to pinpoint the diagnosis. These will show whether there is osteoarthritis of the spine, or a reduction of the spaces between the vertebrae (which means reduction of the intervertebral disk), or a slipped disk (wedge-shaped) which may be impinging on nerves. X-rays will also show whether a growth or tumor is present, that might be pressing on the nerves.

In rare instances, an opaque liquid is injected into the spinal cord so that the exact location of an impingement on a nerve root becomes visible on the X-ray. Exercises are not recommended for anyone with this unfortunate condition, since some of them may produce pain and make matters worse. In any event, any exercises for lower back problems, other than those done weekly as a preventive measure, should be eased into gently to avoid pain.

STRENGTHENING THE ABDOMINAL MUSCLES

☐ Strengthening of the abdominal muscles has already been described in chapter 9. Abdominal muscles are exercised when exhaling—pulling the stomach in and thereby pushing the diaphragm up. You place the strongest demand on the abdominal muscles when you do sit-ups, raising yourself from a lying-down position to a sitting position.

I repeat here an earlier caution in connection with the sit-ups. It happens that the hip flexors are mechanically in a good position to accomplish the first step in allowing us to raise ourselves toward a sitting position. But when the hip flexors are exercised strongly in a lying-down position, unless there are strong abdominal muscles stabilizing the lumbar spine, these vertebrae will end up curving inward with a sudden motion (fig. 47). This is the worst thing that can happen for someone with lower back trouble. Those with weak abdominal muscles and a potential for lower back trouble should start exercising in the following way.

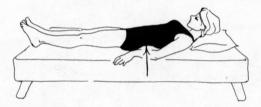

47. *Avoid hollow lower back (lumbar spine).*

• Sitting on the edge of a table, as in knee-swinging, tilt your upper body slowly backward as far as it will go, and then forward again. Make sure that your pelvis is tucked under—the opposite of the buttocks out —so that when you bend your body backward the lumbar spine is straight (fig. 48). You will notice that from day to day you can bend your torso farther back before moving it forward again.

Exercises for strengthening abdominal muscles, figures 48–50b

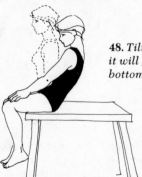

48. *Tilt body back as far as it will go, sit up again (keep bottom tucked under).*

• After about a week of doing the above exercise daily, you can progress to the more difficult exercise. Sit on the bed with knees close to your chest, holding onto your knees with your hands (fig. 49). Swing your torso gently backward as far as it will go without falling, still holding onto your knees, and remain at this point for three seconds (count of six); now sit up straight again. Repeat this as many times as you can until you get tired, each time trying to lean back a little farther. Finally, try to do this without holding on with your hands. Eventually, you will be able to get up from a position in which you are semirecumbent, being propped up with two or three pillows (fig. 50), to the upright sitting position. In time you can reduce the number of pillows, but don't be too ambitious. The best effect in strengthening occurs when the torso is held at about 45 degrees for about three seconds (count of six).

49. Lean backward as far as possible, try to stay a second or two, and sit up again.

50. A little more difficult. Let arms hang down on the side, lean slowly back against the pillows, and sit up again.

Once more: *Never try to get up from a lying down position to a sitting position with an abrupt, jerky movement.* Eventually you will be able to sit up from

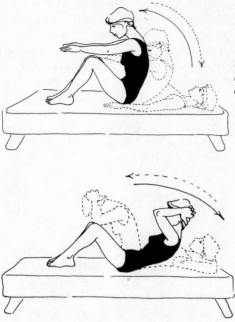

50a. *Now sit up with no pillows behind you. Arms forward make it easier.*

50b. *Do the exercise with hands behind your head. This is the most difficult and the most efficient exercise, to be repeated as often as you can.*

a lying down position with your knees bent (fig. 50a), or even with your hands behind the head (fig. 50b).

You may be wondering how the abdominal muscles, which you can feel contracting at the front of your abdomen, contribute to stabilizing the spinal column, which is at the back. The answer is that the lower spine is not equipped with any muscles anteriorly (forward); posteriorly (in the back), a variety of short and long muscles are directly attached to various vertebrae. These muscles curve the lower spine inward. To press it outward, in order for it to form a straight line, you have to flatten the abdomen so that the only way for the spine to escape is outward. You will get a feeling for this if you sit on a chair and push both forearms against your abdomen; you will feel your spine straightening out. When a heavy girdle is worn, the abdomen is flattened, and the wearer feels more comfortable around the lower spine, since it flattens out posteriorly. A more natural way to get the same effect is to strengthen your abdominal muscles. When strong, they contain the abdomen, just like a strong girdle, and thereby help prevent an exaggerated curve in the spine. When you strengthen your abdominal muscles regularly, their normal length will tend to shorten so that they supply containment for your abdomen without having to be deliberately contracted. If your abdomen has slackened considerably beyond the normal, as happens sometimes after childbirth or after an abdominal operation, do not rely on the above exercises to get you back in shape. Your doctor may prescribe some abdominal support and will advise you when and how much to exercise. One thing is clear: A sagging, bulging abdomen invites lower back problems and requires medical advice.

ISOMETRICS FOR THE ABDOMEN AND LOWER BACK

☐ After you have become aware of how the abdominal muscles feel when they are exercised, you will be able to produce an isometric contraction by pulling the stomach in very strongly and holding it tight for a while, although this is by no means as effective as the exercises described above. This muscle-setting exercise I find particularly helpful for the back muscles, because it is much more convenient to do than the deliberate exercises for those muscles.

• The classic exercise for strengthening the lower back is to lie on the bed on your stomach and raise both legs. If this is not possible at first, raise first one leg a few times, then the other leg (fig. 51) until you can raise both legs slightly off the bed. It is good to use a pillow under the abdomen during this exercise in order not to accentuate the inward curve of the lower spine.

Strengthening the lower back and abdomen, figures 51–55

51. One leg at a time, lift slightly (with a straight knee). Hold for a few seconds.

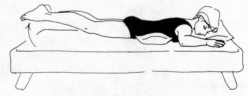

• Another way to strengthen the back muscles is to lie on the bed on your back and raise your knees up, with your feet on the bed. Now, lift your abdomen up to straighten out your hip so that your body forms a straight line between the knees and your chest (fig.

52). Next, lower your buttocks to the bed. Raise and lower a number of times. After several sessions with this exercise, you will become aware of the back muscles, which have to contract in order to raise the body into the desired position.

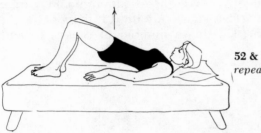

52 & 52a. *Lift buttocks, repeat up to ten times.*

• Here is a final exercise for the abdominal muscles. Lying down with the knees raised (fig. 53), press your lower back firmly against the bed; or standing with the feet placed a few inches out from the wall, flatten the lower back against the wall (fig. 54).

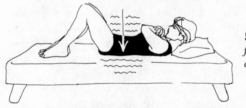

53. *Press lower back flat into bed to the count of six.*

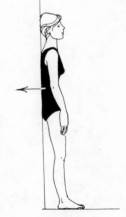

The motion of flattening the back is initiated here by the abdominal muscles, but the back muscles also are tensed to stiffen the lower back as it comes in contact with the surface of the mattress or the wall.

By now you should be able to tense your back muscles and your abdominal muscles at will. It may help you to touch the back muscles during some of these exercises in order to feel what contractions are required to carry through the various motions. This is not easy to accomplish, but it gave me worthwhile feedback.

54. *Press lower back flat against the wall to the count of six.*

STRENGTHENING THE GLUTEALS

☐ Help for lower back trouble also calls for strengthening the buttock muscles. The gluteals, as they are called, are the hip extensors and abductors, moving the legs backward and outward. They are very powerful, voluminous muscles. A frequently cited exercise is to pull the buttock muscles together as strongly as possible and hold the contraction as long as possible. Here is another efficient exercise for the gluteals.

• Lie on the bed with your heels supported on a thick bolster. Now raise your body until it is in a straight line (fig. 55). Do this a number of times, up and down.

55. Raise body in a straight line. Contract buttocks and keep lower back stiff. (Avoid hollow back.) Count to twelve if possible.

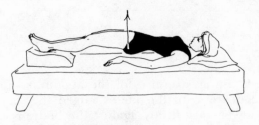

If you have no problem raising yourself ten times, try to raise yourself by supporting yourself only on one heel, with the other heel resting loosely on the bed or held in the air; do not support your body on the other leg. Try to keep your body straight for six seconds (count of twelve). (This exercises both the lower back and the gluteals.) The gluteals are so large that a tensing of at least six seconds seems necessary to achieve a deep contraction of the muscles. At least, that is my experience.

• You can exercise the gluteals while you are sitting on a hard chair by tensing them repeatedly. As you tense them, you feel your body moving up. Hold each contraction as long as six seconds (count of twelve), then relax. Repeat ten to twenty times.

STRENGTHENING THE ABDUCTORS AND ADDUCTORS

☐ The abductor muscles of the legs should also be strengthened with isometric exercises specifically designed for this.

• Sit on the edge of the bed, spreading the legs apart and pushing with your right lower leg against the edge of the bed for six seconds (count of twelve) (fig. 56). Repeat this exercise with the other leg (fig. 57).

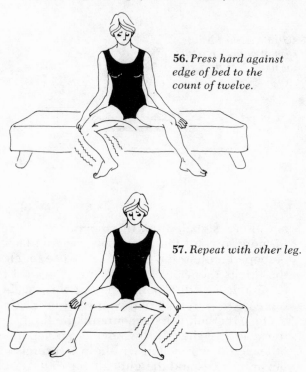

56. *Press hard against
edge of bed to the
count of twelve.*

57. *Repeat with other leg.*

Note that I recommend contracting the abductors for twice as long as other muscles of similar size. This is because the various muscle groups of the thigh are very powerful and hard to isolate. When you attempt to tense them you are unsure of whether you are contracting the desired muscle or another one and so you increase your effort, to obtain a maximum contraction.

• A second way of exercising the abductors is to strain against a leather belt which is looped around the thighs. Do this while you sit on the edge of a bed or a chair. Adjust the belt so that the loop permits your legs to be spread slightly apart. Spread your thighs as forcefully as you can against the leather belt for six seconds (count of twelve) (fig. 58).

Notice that I recommend using a leather belt as a loop rather than an elastic belt, as used with the arms. I find that the elastic belt has too much give for use with the powerful leg muscles; this makes the exercise inefficient. The elastic loop has the advantage of permitting a slight motion, which furnishes

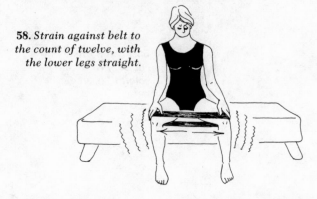

58. *Strain against belt to the count of twelve, with the lower legs straight.*

additional signals from the moving joints, resulting in more forceful muscle action. When a leather belt is looped around the thighs, there is enough give in the thighs themselves as they press against the belt to produce a slight joint motion; this, again, helps increase the strength of the muscle contraction.

Once the belt is looped around the thighs, you can tense against the belt by moving one leg up and the other leg down, which will help to exercise the hip flexor muscles and the gluteals (fig. 59). Reverse the exercise with the other leg (fig. 60).

Exercise hip flexors and gluteals, figures 59 & 60

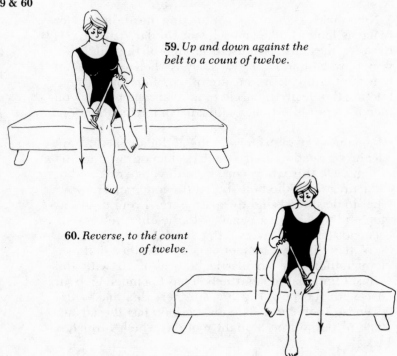

59. *Up and down against the belt to a count of twelve.*

60. *Reverse, to the count of twelve.*

- Still sitting on the edge of a bed or chair, strain thighs against the belt and lower legs with feet rotated inward (fig. 61) and with feet brought together and rotated outward (fig. 62), in order to cover all fibers of the abductor muscles—namely, those that take part in rotating or stabilizing the rotated leg.
- In addition, the abductors may be exercised with the hips straight by straining against the belt while lying down or while standing up.

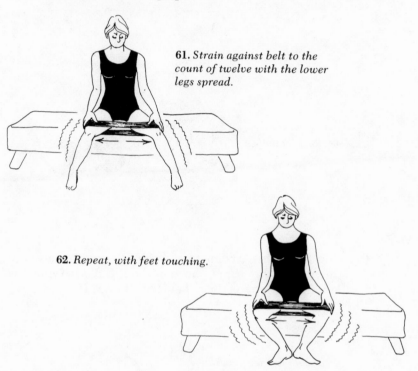

61. *Strain against belt to the count of twelve with the lower legs spread.*

62. *Repeat, with feet touching.*

In the *Royal Canadian Air Force Exercise Manual,* which is in wide use by the general public, hip abductor exercises are stressed especially, since the motions we use in daily life do not strengthen these muscles sufficiently. The RCAF recommends that you lie down on your side and lift your leg into the air as far as you can and as often as you can (fig. 63, right leg; fig. 64, left leg). I found this to be an excellent exercise as long as I did not have a serious hip involvement. If there is hip involvement, the exercise becomes painful and should be avoided.

Pain should not occur during isometric exercises. If it does occur, stop and consider what might be produc-

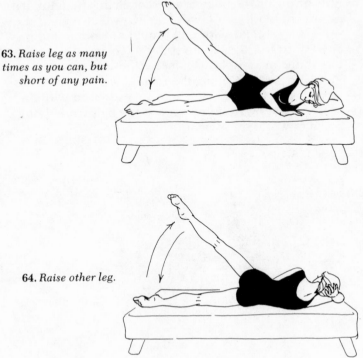

63. *Raise leg as many times as you can, but short of any pain.*

64. *Raise other leg.*

ing the pain. Switch to a different exercise arrangement for the same muscle. You can also practice abducting legs against chair legs (fig. 64a).

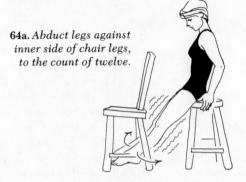

64a. *Abduct legs against inner side of chair legs, to the count of twelve.*

When the abductor muscles of my left hip became extremely weak after extended bed rest and hip involvement, I found the following strengthening procedure most efficient.

• Lie on the bed on your left side with hips at right angles (knees halfway toward chest). Lift the right knee up while the foot still rests on the other leg (fig. 65) and bring it down again. Repeat this as often as you can, with both legs.

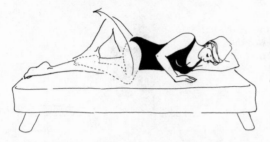

65. *A starter exercise for very weak abductors. Lift right knee as often as you can. Repeat with left knee.*

I could, at first, barely raise the knee once. Repeating it a few times during a single session, I could raise it three times, resting in between. The next day I progressed to ten and later to twenty times. Keeping the foot resting on the opposite lower leg considerably reduces the effort necessary to raise the knee. Once the muscle was sufficiently stimulated with this isotonic exercise, I proceeded to strengthen the abductors isometrically. Before progressing to the belt exercise, I gave resistance in the direction of abduction with both hands.

• Using both hands you can also provide good resistance for exercising adductor muscles. Sit, with your legs spread apart, on a chair or on the edge of a bed. Lean with your hands against your thigh just above the knee (fig. 66). Squeeze your legs together against the resistance of the hands for six seconds (count of twelve). Repeat with other leg.

Strengthening adductors, figures 66–71a

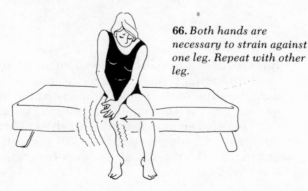

66. *Both hands are necessary to strain against one leg. Repeat with other leg.*

• A different way to exercise the adductor muscles is to squeeze a beach ball between your legs (fig. 67) as hard as possible for six seconds (count of twelve). Repeat with the feet farther apart (fig. 68), and again with the feet placed side by side (fig. 69).

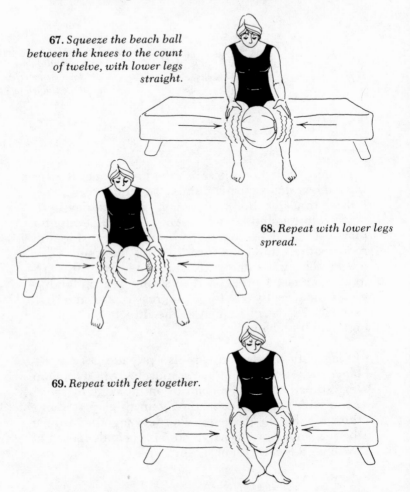

67. *Squeeze the beach ball between the knees to the count of twelve, with lower legs straight.*

68. *Repeat with lower legs spread.*

69. *Repeat with feet together.*

• It is also useful to exercise the adductor muscles with the hips straight. Stand before the edge of an open door, holding on to both doorknobs, and adduct first one leg and then the other leg, pressing it against the door for six seconds (count of twelve). This can be done with the hip extended (fig. 70) and with the hip flexed (fig. 71). You can also adduct legs against chair legs (fig. 71a).

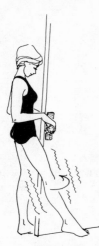

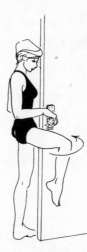

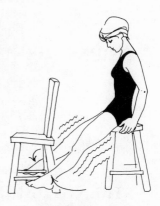

70. *Squeeze leg against door to the count of twelve. Repeat with other leg.*

71. *Squeeze knee against door, to the count of twelve. Repeat with other knee.*

71a. *Adduct legs against outer sides of chair legs, to the count of twelve.*

STRENGTHENING THE HIP FLEXORS

Strengthening the hip flexors, figures 72–74

□ To strengthen the hip flexors, you can provide resistance in various ways at points throughout the range of motion.

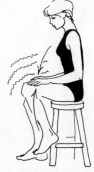

- Raise the thigh against your two resisting hands as in figure 72. You may also bear down on a beach ball as your leg is pressing it up, as in figure 73. Yet another way is to furnish resistance with a leather belt as shown in figure 59.
- When I developed extremely weak hip flexors and abductors on the side of my osteoarthritic hip, my therapist had me slide the leg through its flexion range while I was lying on the other side; the moving leg was supported by a flat board (fig. 74). When I moved my knee toward and away from my chest, I noticed that my heel was riding on the board. In this exercise, the abductor muscle is hardly used and all motion is produced by the hip flexor. The horizontal position and the support of the heel by the board reduce the effective load that the weak hip flexor is called upon to move.

72. *Press leg against both hands to the count of six. Repeat with other leg.*

73. *Press ball down as you raise leg, as hard as you can, to the count of six. Repeat with other leg.*

74. *Draw knee toward chest and back again, several times. The heel may ride on the board. This exercise is meant for very weak flexor muscles.*

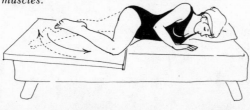

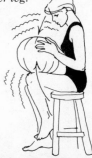

STRENGTHENING THE KNEES

☐ We now turn to strengthening the knee muscles. We are concerned here with the knee extensor, the quadriceps, and the hamstring. For abduction and adduction of the knee, our aim is to strengthen the knee ligaments.

STRENGTHENING THE QUADRICEPS

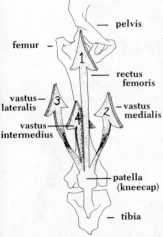

75. The quadriceps helps us to stand upright, to walk, to climb stairs, and to get up from chairs.

☐ Strengthening of the muscles distal and proximal to a joint is of great importance for stabilizing a weakened joint. The muscles distal to the knee are the heel flexors and extensors, which are discussed in chapter 11. Proximal to the knee is the muscle that is usually given the most attention—the quadriceps. As shown in figure 75, this muscle consists of four sections. The longest section originates in the pelvis and passes straight down the front of the thigh; it therefore also acts as a hip flexor, mainly in the first few degrees of raising the leg when we are lying on our back. You can feel this section, no. 1, rectus femoris, contract as you raise the leg; therefore, leg raising from the horizontal position of the body with the knees straight is an exercise that strengthens this muscle (fig. 76). Actually, keeping the leg raised just one or two inches (2.5 to five centimeters) above the bed as long as possible is a good way of strengthening this section. You can also tense (set) the muscle without raising the leg (fig. 77).

Strengthening the quadriceps, figures 76–80

76. *Straight leg raises, as many as possible, first one leg, then the other. This strengthens the rectus femoris.*

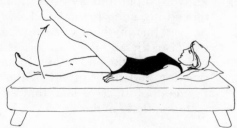

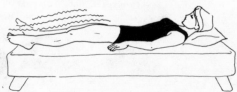

77. *Tense thigh hard to the count of twelve. Repeat with other thigh. Do as often as you can.*

The other three sections are called "vasti." No. 2, the vastus medialis, originates on the inner side of the femur bone; no. 3, the vastus lateralis, originates on the outer side of the femur bone; no. 4, the vastus intermedius, originates on the anterior side of the femur bone. All three, together with the rectus femoris, join in a tendon which is attached to the tibia (shinbone). In this tendon there is embedded the patella (kneecap), a useful mechanical device which increases the efficiency of the various sections of the quadriceps in various positions of flexion of the knee.

There are several ways of strengthening the powerful quadriceps, and it does need strengthening in every arthritic. It is exercised when we walk and climb, for example, and if we curtail such activities it tends to waste. A weak quadriceps results in knee pain as we climb, and so we tend to avoid this more and more and thus a vicious cycle is established.

I would like to describe first one method of strengthening the quadriceps.

• Attach an ankle weight to each ankle. Sit on a table with your legs hanging over the edge; you can place a rolled-up towel under the thighs for comfort. Swing each leg up until it is straight at the knee. Do this as often as you can, first with one leg and then with the other (fig. 78). If you can accomplish this ten times or more, change to a heavier weight, going, say, from two pounds to three pounds, then to five pounds, and so on. (This is a progressive resistance exercise.) Grasp your upper thigh while you swing your leg up. You will notice that the muscle contracts strongly and feels very hard when the leg is all the way up.

An alternative to this exercise is not to swing the

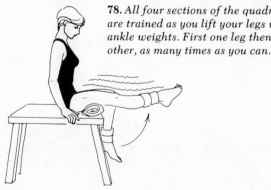

78. *All four sections of the quadriceps are trained as you lift your legs with ankle weights. First one leg then the other, as many times as you can.*

leg, but to hold it out straight, with the ankle weighted down, for as long as possible. (This is an isometric exercise.) If you can last longer than six seconds (count of twelve), you may increase the weight. It is the strong contraction of the quadriceps, not the carrying of the weight per se, that produces the strengthening.

The beautiful thing with the quadriceps is that this is one of the easiest muscles to observe and become aware of its contraction. We can observe it as it contracts at our command, even without any resistance given to the leg. This deliberate muscle contraction, or muscle tensing (setting), should be done as often as possible during the day, each time for six seconds (count of twelve). Contract as forcefully as possible. You can do this muscle setting while sitting in a chair and watching TV, with the knee extended or flexed. You can do it also in bed (fig. 77)—when you wake up in the morning, when you rest during the day, and before you fall asleep.

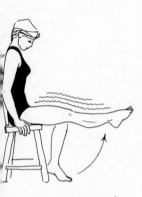

79. *Tense the quadriceps to the count of twelve. You can do this with the knee bent also, but with a straight knee the exercise is more efficient.*

• A more efficient muscle-tensing exercise for the quadriceps is to extend the knee either while sitting or lying down (fig. 79). If the legs are straight, as when you are on the bed, raise them by putting a rolled-up towel under your knees. Extend the knee from the slightly flexed to the straight position (fig. 80). This slight movement of extension displaces the patella to one side, thereby producing better mechanical efficiency for strengthening the various individual parts of the quadriceps.

80. *Tense thigh to the count of twelve, as you straighten the knee. You can do this also without the roll under your knee.*

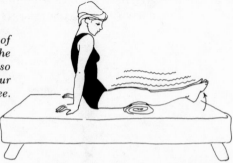

The quadriceps, being equipped with exceptionally long muscle fibers, ideally should be strengthened at various degrees of flexion of the knee. I have described earlier, under stretching of the quadriceps, how you extend the knee from a completely flexed position, using an ankle weight (fig. 40). The same procedure could be done at various degrees of flexion.

In daily life, when you sit on a chair and have in front of you a piece of furniture like a couch, desk, or heavy chair, use it to provide isometric resistance, as if you were trying to lift it up with your foot. The quadriceps is also well exercised every time you get up from a chair. The lower the chair, the more work the quadriceps has to perform. This is good to do, provided you have no hip involvement. Then it is too taxing to try to get up from low chairs, or even from chairs of regular height (fig. 81). In this case you may use a six-inch-high (fifteen-centimeter) seat cushion, Maddak catalogue number H76666, available at surgical supply stores.

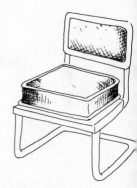

81. *Seat cushion (6" or 15 cm thick) to make it easier to get up from chairs.*

STRENGTHENING THE HAMSTRINGS

☐ The hamstring muscle is the main flexor of the knee and it also extends the pelvis. It is only one-third as powerful as the quadriceps, acting as the antagonist to that muscle. Knee extension is the main function of the knee joint, and the flexor stabilizes this function.

• To exercise the hamstring muscle, flex the knee against resistance. For example, when lying down dig your heels into the bed, with the knees slightly bent (fig. 82). Do this forcefully for three seconds (count of six).

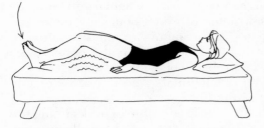

82. *Strengthening the hamstrings. Dig heels into the front edge of the bed or the surface of the bed, as hard as possible to the count of six.*

While sitting down, you can press your heels firmly against the feet of the chair, one at a time. After you have warmed up your hamstring muscles with a few of these isometric exercises, stretch them with one of the exercises mentioned earlier. Stretch-

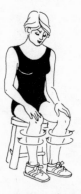

ing of the hamstring may be even more important than strengthening it.

Several muscles help to rotate the leg internally or externally in the bent position; they can be exercised while sitting.

• Press the foot very hard to the floor (preferably while wearing rubber-soled shoes). At the same time, rotate the lower leg to one side as forcefully as possible for three seconds (count of six), and then rotate to the other side (fig. 83).

83. Press foot into ground and rotate the lower leg. Repeat with other foot.

Complementary Exercise

Repeat movements with the other leg.

KEEPING "UP AND AROUND"

☐ The system of exercise I describe in this chapter has helped greatly to keep me fairly mobile, despite instability in one of my hip joints. At first, I was prescribed one cane (to be used on the side opposite the weakened hip). Then, I was prescribed two canes. Later, I was fitted with forearm crutches, which I could not handle because of unstable elbow joints. I finally used a wheelchair when I had to cover distances of more than fifty feet; I was very reluctant to use the wheelchair for shorter distances. My orthopedic surgeon advised me to walk frequently for short distances throughout the day, in order to maintain my ambulation (ability to walk). I foresaw with great concern the day when I might have to use a wheelchair inside my apartment. I saw demonstrations of narrow, motorized wheelchairs that could maneuver around corners and through narrow doors. These are highly sophisticated vehicles, and are probably of great use to persons who cannot be further rehabilitated by hip replacement, such as stroke victims.

For me as an arthritic, being able to walk around the house and garden and across the sidewalk to a taxi represents an acceptable way of life short of a total hip-replacement operation. Exercises during this period are essential to keep the arthritic going in the real sense of the word, since the accustomed brisk walking of former years may now be impossible. In my case, the "arthritis of the hip" is apparently more degenerative (osteoarthritic) rather than rheumatoid in nature. The joint space appears much reduced and the cartilage is largely used up. I have been seen by a number of specialists in the field—orthopedic surgeons, rheumatologists, radiologists, physiatrists, and general practitioners—and hardly any two of these physicians have agreed in their measurement of my disability versus the X-ray findings. The X-rays of both hips seemed remarkably alike, although only one hip was giving me trouble. What they did agree on, however, was the need for regular exercise; they also favor eventual total hip replacement, if life should become unbearable.

I believe that the troublesome hip could have been helped sooner by efficient exercise. But this was prevented by a lower back problem, which caused spasms and muscle weakness on one side. Exercising regularly for both conditions, hip and lower back, has worked out reasonably well to keep me ambulatory within a limited range.

Brisk walking is obviously not possible for someone with severe hip involvement. Furthermore, I was advised by my orthopedic surgeon against an exercise bicycle. I had tried one and observed a slight pain at certain parts of the pedal cycle. In osteoarthritis, you see, one is liable to develop some pain in the capsule of the joint due to the exaggerated stresses of stretching and twisting which result from the abnormal alignment of the joint. We concentrate not only on stretching, but also on strengthening and toning the muscles that govern the motion of the joint.

We cannot figure out every muscle that has to be exercised in order to avoid pain. I have learned from my experience with the hand that it is best to exercise all muscles and let our bodies decide for themselves exactly which muscles they will make use of, so that we can continue to function at the best possible level.

When we suffer some decrease in strength in the upper extremities we can often help ourselves by using both hands and both arms instead of just one to accomplish the desired task. However, we normally require *both* legs to walk. In such a case, we use first one cane and then, if necessary, two canes. But you can do this only if your hands are in good enough shape, and even then you cannot put as much weight onto the canes as a normal person could. The rheumatoid arthritic can lean even less weight on a cane than can an osteoarthritic.

I even made a little experiment to find out how much weight I can take off my bad hip when leaning on canes. I stepped on the bathroom scale and noted my weight. I then leaned first on one cane, and then on both canes, and again marked my weight. I saw that with my right cane I could reduce my body weight by twenty-five pounds; with the second cane my weight came down by another ten pounds. This is a thirty-five-pound reduction, or about one-quarter of my total body weight. You will now easily understand why your doctor may tell you to lose ten pounds; in my case it would be the equivalent of using one cane.

I made the same test with a person in normal good health. We found that he could reduce his body weight by thirty-five pounds *with each cane.* So, you see, we rheumatoid arthritics are quite handicapped in this respect.

Fortunately, today excellent results are being achieved with total hip-replacement surgery. In this operation, the head of the femur is replaced by a metal ball that is rooted in the core of the femur bone. A plastic receptacle that functions like the acetabulum is attached to the pelvis (see figure 3). Both artificial parts are secured with plastic cement. At the present time this operation is postponed until the level of discomfort demands it. It will be some years before the long-term effects of the procedure are fully evaluated. It is not known, for example, how long the replacement remains satisfactorily cemented to the bones or whether infection is likely to develop indicating removal of the artificial joint. The whole procedure is not yet twenty years old, and doctors prefer not to subject their younger patients to this drastic measure in case it proves to be something less than permanent.

When our knees and hips become arthritic, we have trouble flexing these joints simultaneously in order to put on our socks and shoes. You may find the following self-help devices useful: long shoehorns; elastic shoe-laces, which permit shoes to be slipped on or off without being tied or untied; a sock aid, a contraption to help you to pull your socks on (available from surgical supply stores).

There are a variety of so-called reachers available to permit one to pick up objects from the floor without having to bend down. Some of these are intricate me-

chanical devices and require a degree of manual ability. If your hands are seriously involved, try out the
device at a surgical supply store before you buy one.

Note: For information about how you can obtain the
devices and special equipment mentioned in this
chapter, consult the Directory of Aids.

11 Saturday Night: Feet and Ankles

☐ Few of us in our lives require the degree of foot and ankle flexibility exhibited by the ballet dancer, who is able to balance her body on the toes of one foot while holding her ankle completely straight (fig. 1). Yet even in ordinary locomotion we, too, exhibit a remarkable flexibility. When we walk our feet and ankles are flexing to compensate for any unevenness of the ground and for the weight of the body as it bears down first on one foot, then on the other.

1. Support total body weight on the toes of one foot.

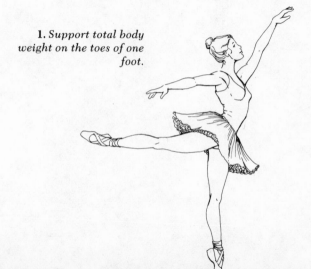

If we lose flexibility in our feet and ankles we begin to appreciate how important they are to the task of supporting and balancing the body. We find it difficult to stand and move steadily; our feet cannot easily conform to the ground, with the result that there may be undue stress on the hips and knees, leading to degenerative osteoarthritis. So it is very important to maintain this flexibility as well as we can.

THE STRUCTURE OF THE FOOT

☐ When we walk or jump, the impact on our feet is absorbed largely by the two flexible arches of the foot, the transverse (metatarsal arch) and the longitudinal arch (figs. 2a, 2b), and by the muscles of the ankle.

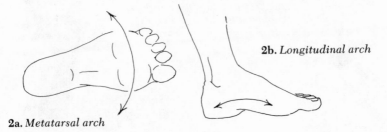

2b. *Longitudinal arch*

2a. *Metatarsal arch*

After the foot hits the ground, the ankle tends to bend slightly and then straighten out. The same thing occurs at the knee, where the powerful flexors and extensors absorb part of the impact. The hip, however, receives the full force of the remaining impact, since we usually do not flex and extend the hip as much as we do the joints of the extremities. (This may be the reason why in many cases the hip is the first area to exhibit degenerative osteoarthritic changes.)

To better understand the foot exercises and supports that I describe in this chapter, a little biomechanical and anatomical discussion of the feet is in order.

Anatomically, the feet and the hands are similar, except that the sizes of the individual elements are different. Instead of the *carpal* bones of the hand, we have the much larger *tarsal* bones of the feet. The largest one, the calcaneus, forms the heel; attached to this bone is the powerful Achilles tendon, which is pulled by the calf muscles in order to flex the foot.

Forward of the tarsal bones are the five *metatarsal* bones, similar to the *metacarpal* bones of the hand. The metatarsal bones are joined to the phalanges of the five toes, forming the metatarsal phalangeal joints (MTP), which correspond to the metacarpal phalangeal joints (MCP) of the hands. The MTP joints are linked in the flexible metatarsal arch that is held together by strong transverse ligaments.

During a walking stroke, the heel normally strikes the ground first, followed by the outside of the sole. Next, the metatarsal arch touches the ground, and finally the toes push off to propel you forward (fig. 3). The points of contact with the ground can be observed by looking at a footprint (fig. 4).

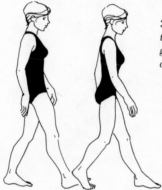

3. *During the walking stroke, the heel strikes first against the ground. Finally the toes push off to propel you forward.*

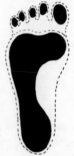

4. *The footprint indicates contact with the ground: heel, outside edge of foot, ball of foot, and toes.*

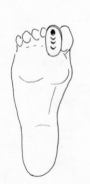

5. *Splint to spread toes*

In rheumatoid arthritis, the MTP joints of the feet are subject to attack and deformities result that are similar to those in the MCP joints of the hands. The ulnar deviation of the fingers is paralleled in the foot by the big toe turning toward the other toes. This may cause a bunion to form at the MTP joint of the big toe. The other toes are held in place by the outside edge of the shoe. (The design of a pointed shoe actually forces the big toe into this unnatural position, from which it normally can be rescued by toe-spreading exercises, unless the MTP joint of the big toe has been damaged and the extensor tendon has slipped off the joint.) When the big toe deviates in this way it cannot contribute much strength to push-off at the end of the walking stroke. A splint is available from Dr. Scholl to spread the big toe back again (fig. 5).

I have begun by emphasizing the importance of flexibility because only one out of ten physicians I've talked to has ever brought up this subject. Physicians usually are satisfied if they can make out the proper prescription to alleviate the pain or discomfort of the patient. In case of foot problems, the "sure to work" prescriptions are proper shoes with supports for the longitudinal arches and a metatarsal pad (usually the longitudinal arch support is molded individually). Later, supports are changed as necessary and wider shoes are prescribed as the foot slowly spreads, due to depressed arches. Eventually a molded shoe is called for, and finally an operation on the front part of the foot may be indicated. The fact that exercise and massage can help to keep the foot flexible and strong, and thereby extend the time until more radical measures or prescriptions are required, is rarely mentioned.

I hope my readers will find the exercises and other measures I describe as helpful as I have found them to be.

THE METATARSAL ARCH

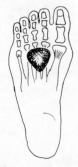

6. *Insert in shoe. Metatarsal pad, located just behind the metatarsal joint*

□ Orthopedic surgeons usually look at the sole of your shoe to observe the pattern of wear. By comparing this with normal patterns of wear, they can judge what supports and exercises are required in any particular case. If the tip of a shoe is not worn, then push-off is taking place at the metatarsal arch. This overloads the already vulnerable arch and may further stretch the transverse ligament, so that eventually the arch collapses.

The normal action of the intact metatarsal (transverse) arch is to absorb part of the shock in walking or jumping. The arch flattens out momentarily like a spring and then resumes its original shape. Once the arch "falls," meaning that it no longer springs back to its original shape, it should be supported by a metatarsal pad installed in shoe and placed directly behind the arch (fig. 6). If you do not use such a support you're liable to experience pain and further deterioration (if you have rheumatoid arthritis) of the metatarsal arch, with the result that the toes will ride up (fig. 7). The toe that is then elevated will rub painfully against the shoe and become inefficient in pushing off during walking. The shoe will no longer show a pattern of wear at its tip.

The exact size and placement of metatarsal pads de-

7. *Toe "riding up" due to damaged metatarsal joint*

pends on the individual foot. If you have not been prescribed full-length supports as yet—including metatarsal supports—you may experiment by inserting metatarsal pads (available, for instance, from Dr. Scholl) in your shoes, moving them around until you find the most comfortable position just behind the arch.

Early use of metatarsal pads will do much to prevent the toes from riding up.

STRENGTHENING THE TOES

Isometric strengthening of toes, figures 8–11

□ To restore needed power to the toes for correct push-off, the toes can be strengthened individually with isometric exercises.

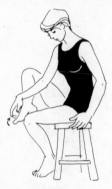

8. *Push toes against fingers, one at a time.*

• Offer resistance to the tip of each toe; you can use a finger for this or something like the edge of a book (figs. 8, 9).
• Isometric strengthening of the toes, in various directions, can be done inside the shoe. While sitting, spread the toes apart against the sides of the shoe to the count of six. Extend the toes upward against the resistance of the shoe to a count of six. Press the toes against the sole of the shoe to a count of six.
• Curling the toes is also very helpful. A good exercise is to pick up a pencil with the toes or grasp a washcloth with the toes and pull against resistance (figs. 10, 11).
• The toes also should be spread and extended upward as far as possible as a range-of-motion exercise (fig. 12).

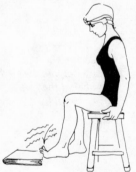

9. *Push toes against the edge of a book.*

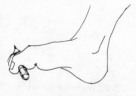

11. *Grasp a washcloth and pull it between feet.*

ıp a pencil.

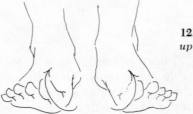

12. *Spread and extend toes upward as far as possible.*

I eventually had to use splints at night to spread the big toes (fig. 5), and after a month or two of this, I found I was able to exert more control over the big toe in spreading exercises. I noticed that if I stopped wearing the splints at night and did not do any spreading exercises, the big toe tended to wander underneath the second toe (fig. 7). Such a complication should be avoided by all means, if possible.

MAINTAINING THE LONGITUDINAL ARCH

☐ Orthopedic correction of the longitudinal arches is important in keeping rheumatoid arthritic feet properly aligned and in preventing damage to other joints, such as knees and hips. However, it can easily be seen that if the longitudinal, as well as the metatarsal arches are fully and solidly supported, all "springiness" is taken out of the foot. This should be countered by exercise and massage to help prevent atrophy and tightness in the muscles.

Here is an exercise to strengthen the longitudinal arch.

• Walk on the outside of your feet (fig. 13). At first do this for a few steps, then try to increase the number of steps until you can walk this way for a minute or so. Do the exercise in the course of the day with or without shoes.

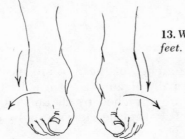

13. *Walk on the outside of the feet.*

MIND OVER MUSCLE

☐ Eventually, I have obtained enough feedback from my feet to enable me to tense the muscles involved in walking on the outside of the feet without actually doing the walking, just like flexing the biceps. If someone had told me years ago to contract these particular muscles deliberately, I would have laughed at the idea. However, I now know from experience that when I make myself aware of the contraction of muscles anywhere in the body in the course of walking, or using the arms, or whatever activity, I can learn to contract these muscles at will. Most muscles send out sufficiently strong signals so that you can become aware of how they are acting. With practice you can learn to contract or relax them at will. This is not a mental process in the usual sense of the word. It involves the use of a "sixth sense," the proprioceptive sense, which deals with signals emanating from within your body. In order to develop this sense you have to exclude everything else and concentrate on what you wish to accomplish. This is similar to biofeedback control of blood pressure and heartbeat, except that becoming aware of our muscles and actuating them at will is a simpler process and does not require the use of any electronic aids.

See if you can become aware of your muscles acting in the following exercise, also for the longitudinal arch.

• Place the foot on the floor in as flatfooted a position as possible. Then try to raise the arch of the foot by tensing your muscles, but without raising the heel or toe from the floor. Do this ten times at each session, and you probably will become aware of these muscles and will be able to exercise them several times during the course of a day, inside your shoe.

USING SUPPORTS

☐ Since the arches of the foot are basically held in their position by ligaments, it can be assumed that once these are stretched by rheumatoid arthritis the only course is to replace their action by rigid or cushioned supports, which act as splints. In my own case, I prefer to put the emphasis on keeping the muscles strong and flexible. Indeed, the one physician who told me to exercise my feet told me at the same time not to wear rigid supports, since they would tend to stiffen my foot muscles.

Nevertheless, there are times when I absolutely need the support of rigid corrective arches. This would be the case after long periods of immobilization.

Once, after prolonged bed rest (which was not connected with arthritis), I found that my feet had become so weak I could not maintain the longitudinal arch; I was walking flatfooted with toes pointing outward. This, in turn, threw my knees out of alignment, producing intense pain.

Early examinations suggested arthritic changes in the knee which might require an operation. After a year or so of struggling, I saw my orthopedic surgeon, who diagnosed the problem as coming from the feet. He prescribed a type of corrective arch support developed at the University of California at Berkeley. The Berkeley support consists of a molded plastic shell that surrounds the foot, maintaining it in the position that the technician has found to provide the best alignment of the entire structure of the leg (fig. 14). The shell is molded from a plaster cast taken while the foot is held at the correct angle. Walking with these Berkeley insoles was somewhat painful in the beginning; at every step, some of the muscles and ligaments in the feet get stretched. However, the result was excellent in dramatically removing all pain from my knees.

I firmly believe I could have avoided having to correct my feet with the Berkeley insoles if I had been more conscious of the mechanics and requirements of the feet and had spent a little time one evening each week on them, maintaining flexibility and strength. My time for the feet now is Friday evening. Now after any period of immobilization, as soon as some muscle strength is regained (that is, as soon as I can walk a few steps barefoot without too much pain), I start on a deliberate program of muscle strengthening. At the same time, I make use of arch supports of a springy material that permits the foot to exercise while walking.

I hope it is clear from the foregoing that exercising for flexibility and strength alone, as we do for the other

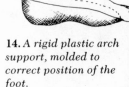

14. *A rigid plastic arch support, molded to correct position of the foot.*

joints of the body, is not sufficient for the feet and ankles. We have to adjust our approach to meet each new situation, which often means splinting in the form of arch supports and always the selection of proper shoes.

PROPER SHOES ARE A MUST

☐ Your rheumatologist probably will have told you to be sure to wear comfortable shoes. Once you need arch supports, either for the longitudinal arch or the metatarsal arch or both, you may be referred to an orthopedic surgeon who will prescribe the type of support and correction needed, and recommend an arch support source. He probably will tell you to wear these supports in low-heeled oxford-type shoes, with as many eyelets as possible, and firm soles. These specifications are designed to keep the raised portions for the arch support and your foot correctly engaged at all times. (I have found that as long as I did not need very strong correction for the metatarsal arch, I could get away with soft-soled shoes. Later, however, when I needed rather a large support pad for the metatarsal, I noticed that in the push-off phase of the gait, my toes would bend and my foot would slip forward, away from the metatarsal support. This was painful and so I returned to the stiffer sole, which prevented the foot from curling up in the push-off phase.)

Both the orthopedic shoemaker who prepared the support and the orthopedic surgeon who checked on the proper fit of the supports and shoes observed how the sole was wearing. If the fit is correct, the sole should show wear near the outer edge and under the ball of the foot as well as the tip. If this is not the case, the experts will suggest some change in the support.

It would seem that after you insert a metatarsal support of the right size at just the right spot, you're guaranteed to be free of pain and callouses in this area. Unfortunately, I've found that the pads are not 100 percent efficient. When we take a step and the heel, followed by the metatarsal arch, strikes the ground, the longitudinal arch acts like a spring and flattens out slightly, thereby absorbing shock (fig. 15). As the longitudinal arch flattens, the metatarsal arch area and the toes move slightly forward in the shoe while the heel remains in place. This is why we select shoes that give

15. *The longitudinal arch
flattens slightly during
walking.*

some space in front of our toes. Our toes move forward
and back in the shoe as we walk. The metatarsal support, however, is stationary in the shoe. Thus, the metatarsal area of the foot glides beyond the metatarsal
pad during walking, bringing the metatarsal heads
closer to the sole of the shoe, particularly during the
last part of the stride (fig. 15). The result is often pain
and callouses. If this condition cannot be contained,
an operation is sometimes performed to remove the
heads of the metatarsal bones, the so-called forefoot
operation, which is usually expected to result in great
benefit.

HEAT, MASSAGE, AND HYDROTHERAPY
FOR THE FEET

☐ Some words about heat and massage. As we have
learned with other joints of the body it is beneficial to
relax muscles before exercising them. This can be
done, as I've described, by tensing muscles, then relaxing them and repeating this sequence a few times
before extending the joint's exercise range. I will
come back to this in more detail describing exercises
for the ankle.

For the foot proper, heat and massage provide a
pleasant relaxation before exercise. Try dissolving
some commercial foot-bath powders in a hot foot bath.
Your feet will come out wonderfully relaxed. These
powders usually contain salicylates, basically aspirin,
to increase circulation.

An excellent way to relax the muscles of the feet is
the whirlpool bath; most podiatrists (foot doctors) have

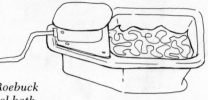

16. *A small Sears, Roebuck*
     whirlpool bath.

facilities for this. Circulation is increased by immersing the feet in the whirlpool for ten to twenty minutes. You'll find that you can withstand very hot water in a whirlpool. The massaging action of the swirling water increases circulation, which dissipates heat away from the surface of the skin and prevents the foot from overheating.

I bought a small whirlpool bath (fig. 16) from Sears, Roebuck which I find useful for hands, elbows, feet, and ankles. Fifteen minutes in the whirlpool bath leave my feet refreshed and decrease the pain, probably because the bath removes stagnating lymph from around joints. After such a bath I feel much more inclined to spread and curl the toes, walk on the outside of my feet and rotate my ankles.

I hope you will keep in mind that constant muscular action and motion is necessary to dissipate lymph from the feet, especially when you are upright and fluids tend to pool in the extremities. At night, too, there is a tendency for the circulation of the lymphatic fluid in the feet to become sluggish. You wake up in the morning with your feet very slightly swollen. When you put your slippers on and walk around a bit you dissipate the fluids and your walking shoes then will fit you much better.

It is important for arthritics to realize this, because their movement is somewhat restricted and they tend to accumulate fluid in their feet. For this reason, I sometimes in the course of the day do a vibrating exercise with my foot and leg, especially after sitting for a long period of time. With the toes resting on the ground, I flex the calf muscle to produce a rapid up and down pumping motion of the heel and knee.

Professional massage of the feet, especially oriental massage, has a very invigorating effect. This is usually part of a total body massage. Foot muscles can be loosened up much more than with whirlpool massage, and joints that tend to get out of alignment can be realigned, at least temporarily, to prevent stiffening at bad angles. Such a massage is quite a luxurious thing, but rather expensive, and therefore cannot be enjoyed by most routinely.

A good exercise with a massaging effect is walking barefoot on a sandy beach, especially when the sand is warm. Walking in loose, dry sand exercises every single muscle of the foot, as the foot adjusts to the uneven surface.

I have found that rolling the sole of the foot back and forth firmly over a small rubber ball or a tennis ball imitates a massage action (fig. 17). I recommend this highly for your weekly evening foot and ankle exercise session, especially if you wear firm longitudinal arch supports, which tend to make the feet stiff.

The Chinese long ago recognized the importance of the feet to the total health of the body. Indeed, their method of acupressure on various parts of the soles is supposed to have a healing effect on such organs as the heart, lungs, and liver. Whether there is any truth to this is doubtful, but I do share the belief that the health of the entire skeletal system benefits when the feet are kept supple. I have noticed that if I experience pain in my feet while walking—let us say due to a painful metatarsal arch—I tend to pull my shoulders up and my neck becomes stiff.

17. *Rolling a ball beneath the foot provides massage action.*

THE ANKLES

☐ Twisting an ankle can happen to anyone. Almost everyone has had the experience at one time or another, and we know that it can be quite painful. With someone in normal good health, the pain usually goes away within a few days. Unfortunately, after I contracted rheumatoid arthritis, I found that twisting an ankle became a much more serious problem. It happened more frequently and then the pain did not go away in a few days; sometimes it lingered on through the whole winter. As in most cases of pain around joints, this pain comes from excessive strain on a ligament. The muscles are weak or underused, and too much resiliency is expected from the ligament.

Exercising the muscles around the ankle is one way to make sure that the range of motion of the ankle is preserved. In this way, we stretch the muscles to at least their normal length and keep them working efficiently. By strengthening the muscles, we ensure that the stability of the joint does not depend solely on ligaments, which become vulnerable in rheumatoid arthritis.

TESTING THE ANKLE RANGES

☐ Before doing ankle exercises, it is useful to take a warm whirlpool bath if you have any swelling.

• First let's check our ranges. Keeping the heel on the floor, extend the toes up toward the knee as far as possible. This will extend the ankle. You should be able to reach at least ninety degrees (fig. 18).

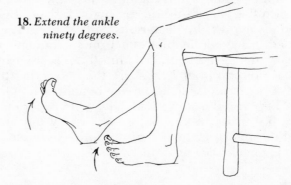

18. *Extend the ankle ninety degrees.*

• Next, flex the outstretched ankle by leaving the heel on the floor (fig. 19). You do not have to try to form a straight line with your leg and foot. A somewhat shorter range will be sufficient for the requirements of daily life.

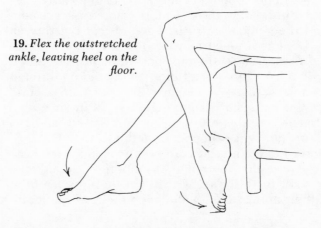

19. *Flex the outstretched ankle, leaving heel on the floor.*

• Next, rotate the feet outward (abduct) as far as possible, keeping the heels on the floor. Then, rotate them inward (adduct) (fig. 20).

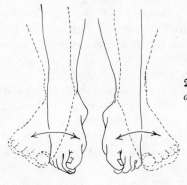

20. *Rotate feet outward and inward.*

• Next, bend the ankles as far as possible so that the feet rest on their outer edges (inversion of the feet). Now do it the other way, moving the ankles all the way in the opposite direction so that the feet rest on the inner edges of the soles of the feet (eversion of the feet).
• Finally, circle each foot, always keeping the heel on the floor and the toes raised (fig. 21).

In this manner go through all the ranges. Start with the ankle extended and the toes all the way up; flex the ankle and point toes downward; rotate the feet outward and inward with heels on the floor; invert feet so that they rest on outer edges of soles, then evert the feet so that they rest on the inner edges of the soles; finally, circle each foot in opposite directions (fig. 21).

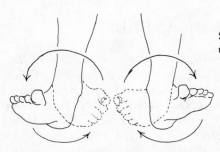

21. *Circle each foot with heels on the floor.*

If no pain or hesitation of motion is experienced while doing these exercises the ranges are probably all right and it is sufficient exercise for you to go through the ranges of motion a few times. If you are not satisfied with your performance, repeat the sequence after exercising all the muscles of the ankle by tensing them (holding the ankle very stiff, as though resisting a strong load in all directions simultaneously). You will get a better feel for this contraction after you have done some isometric exercises against resistance. Pressing the sole or the upper part of your foot strongly against the rung of a chair or table will make you aware of the muscles on the side of the shinbone and in the calf as well as those in the ankle. Different muscles are contracted when you lift your toes up (the muscles on the side of the shinbone) and when you press your toes to the floor (the muscles of the calf). To hold the ankle entirely stiff, you contract all these various muscles. This warms them up and makes them more flexible, especially if you tense and relax them several times in a row. Now you will be able to achieve more when you exercise your ranges.

If you work with a therapist, he or she may set up resistance to movement of the foot in one direction and then, after relaxation, move the foot in the opposite direction. This is the classical PNF, or proprioceptive neuromuscular facilitation, exercise (hold-relax technique) which I have modified in this system of exercise by substituting muscle tensing or voluntary contraction for the contraction against the resisting hand of the therapist (tense-relax-and-stretch technique). If you have had the opportunity to do this exercise once with a therapist, it will then be easier for you to carry it out on your own in a regular home routine.

ISOMETRICS FOR THE ANKLES

□ The positions of the feet for isometric exercises closely follow the positions used in the range-of-motion exercises. The only difference is that the isometric exercises strengthen certain muscles. For instance, by extending the ankle (pointing the feet up), you stretch the calf muscles and *strengthen* the muscles on the shinbone of the leg. You can feel them contract if you press them with your fingers as you lift your foot.

• The type of resistance to use for the isometric exercises can be left to your own choice. The main thing to remember is that you exercise your feet up and down (extension and flexion); and laterally to the outside and the inside (external and internal rotation). Do each contraction with maximum effort for three seconds (count of six).

One set of muscles requires special attention. These are the very powerful calf muscles, which help us push off when we walk or run. It is not so simple to find the appropriate resistance for these muscles. The following exercise, however, is helpful.

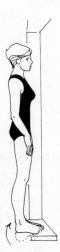

22. *Stand with the front part of feet on doorsill and raise heels.*

• Stand with the front part of your feet on the doorsill and lift your heels up (fig. 22). Repeat this up to twenty times, up and down. As you gain strength in your calves try to lift yourself up on the front part of one foot only, so the whole body weight is on that foot, then do the same on the other foot. You will become aware of the tensing of these muscles, so that when you want to contract them voluntarily in a muscle-setting exercise you will be able to do so. You should do this a few times during the day, especially if you do not take vigorous walks anymore. Remember that the calf muscles help to stabilize both the knees and the ankles and are therefore very important in maintaining good strength. Eventually you will be able to walk on tiptoes, and finally to stand on the toes of one foot for three seconds (count of six).
• To strengthen the ankles in other directions, I have found it helpful to extend them by raising the front part of the foot against the bottom edge of a couch or the lower rung of a heavy table, keeping my heels on the floor. You can feel the muscles contracting on your shinbone when you do this.
• Next, you abduct and adduct the feet against resistance. First, press hard with the outer edge of the front part of the foot against the leg of a piece of furniture. Contract for three seconds (count of six), and relax. Then press the chair or table leg with the inside of the forefoot. Contract for three seconds (count of six), and relax. Do the same sequence with the other foot.

• Finally, walk twenty paces on the outer edge of your soles (fig. 23). This is a specific exercise to strengthen important ankle and calf muscles.

23. Walk twenty paces on outer edges of soles to strengthen the ankle and calf muscles.

After doing these exercises a number of times you should become aware of how the ankle feels when it is held stiffly. The ankle has to be very firm and stiff in order to withstand the pressure of abducting and adducting it forcefully against the chair or table leg. Having become aware of how a stiff ankle feels, you may practice muscle tensing of the ankles without external resistance.

ACT AT THE FIRST SIGN OF PAIN

☐ Before I contracted arthritis, I played football and did some mountain climbing. Such activities strengthened the ankles. Even walking briskly helps. When you cannot do these things anymore, deliberate exercises are necessary to maintain the strength of the ankle and to avoid damaging the ligaments. Once an ankle is twisted or merely feels painful, I wrap it in an Ace bandage (follow the instructions on the package or have your therapist explain how to wrap the bandage around the ankle). Sometimes it has helped just to have the Ace bandage on overnight. I think we only harm ourselves by trying to tough it out and disregard the pain. Respect the pain, and try to rid yourself of it with whatever measures are available to you—heat, massage, wrapping and/or whirlpool bath. And in doing your range-of-motion exercises, stop short of causing pain.

Note: For information about how you can obtain the devices and special equipment mentioned in this chapter, consult the Directory of Aids.

The Daily Five-Minute Tense-Relax-and- Stretch Routine 12

□ This may be the most important chapter of this book. It is placed here at the end so that you can go to it quickly. You now have achieved a degree of body awareness and have learned about the crippling aspects of arthritis and how exercises can play a preventive role. I do not mean that you can avoid arthritis altogether, but as long as you do your daily stretching exercises, you can very often delay the onset of crippling symptoms and maintain flexibility.

I prefer to spend no more than five minutes on these daily stretching sessions; once the motions are internalized, you can repeat individual ones in the course of the day. For instance, when reaching for a jar on an upper shelf (fig. 1), be aware that you are repeating an important stretch motion. Reach also with the other arm to complete this part of the exercise. After sitting for a while in a chair and before getting up, tense your quadriceps muscles first on one thigh and then on the other. When you get up from a lying position remember to tense the abdominal muscles deliberately as you perform the motion. When you sit on a chair, cross your legs occasionally to exercise your hip range (fig. 2). Make it a custom to take a few deliberate deep breaths during the day, and while you are going for a walk always remember to maintain a good posture. As

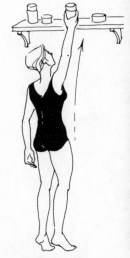

1. *Stretch while reaching for a jar.*

255

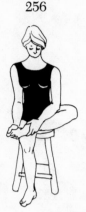

2. *When sitting on a chair, cross your legs occasionally to exercise your hip range.*

long as it does not represent a strain for you, walk briskly for at least ten minutes a day to stimulate your cardiovascular system and maintain your leg muscles. In the course of the day, do isometric exercises for the quadriceps, pressing upward with your foot against a heavy piece of furniture, or sideways to exercise the abductors or any other muscles which you feel need a little extra attention. Squeeze your buttocks together as hard as possible once or twice a day. After you brush your teeth in the morning or evening, while standing in front of the bathroom mirror, gargle and observe how far back you can bend your head. Even if you do not customarily gargle, bend your head back all the way, then go through the various ranges of the motion of the head, leaning it forward and sideways, and rotating it left and right. When you sit at your desk, grasp a pencil occasionally between the phalanges of your fingers to maintain finger flexibility (fig. 3). When you sit, try not to keep your legs together but instead hold them slightly apart.

3. *Sitting at a desk, grasp a pencil between the phalanges, as shown, with the large knuckles straight.*

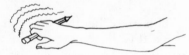

PREPARATION

☐ The best time to do the daily five-minute tense-relax-and-stretch exercise routine is definitely in the morning, when it will help you to become fully awake and limber. You may have observed cats stretching themselves after waking up. They have a good reason for this, and we can follow their example.

If you suffer from morning stiffness and are able to take a warm bath, then do the exercises right after the bath. Some of them can even be done while you are in the bathtub. For instance, you can stretch your gluteals, quadriceps, and hamstrings by bringing the knees close to the chest, grasping the underside of the thigh first with the knee bent and then with the knee straight and pulling the leg toward your chest, and finally grasping your shinbone with the knee bent.

Stretching the arms and neck is easy to do while you are taking a shower; the shoulder and neck area is warmed up and massaged by the jet of water, and the pipe connecting the shower head is convenient for an upward reach with your hands.

When you leave the bathroom and return to your bedroom to exercise, be sure that you don't get chilled. Avoid drafts and try to have your bedroom temperature at least 72° F (22° C). Now you are really ready for the five-minute workout. Your body is nicely warmed up and will permit the muscles to be stretched with a minimum of effort to the limit of their possible ranges.

If you do not take a bath in the morning, you can do the exercises soon after you wake up. Remember, you may be a little bit stiff, so you should do some isometric muscle setting for each limb to warm it up before moving through the full range of motion. Do the exercises on a firm bed, preferably with only a small pillow under your head. Have the window at least slightly open so that you breathe easier, but *do not get chilled.* Here goes.

THE EXERCISES

- Yawn heartily once or twice, then open your mouth briefly as wide as you can (fig. 4).
- Lying on your back, inhale once or twice deeply as you have learned in chapter 9, on breathing. First, fill the upper area of your lungs with air, then the middle part and finally the lower part, by pushing the stomach out. Exhale completely each time by first pulling the stomach in and then pulling the rib cage in.

  It is good to fill your lungs this way with fresh air coming in from the open window. We have replenished our oxygen and stimulated our circulation and are ready for the next step.
- Lying on your back, stretch your arms overhead (fig. 5) and tense as strongly as possible all the muscles in

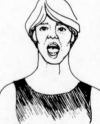

4. Yawn heartily, relax, and then open your mouth as wide as possible.

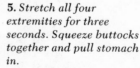

5. Stretch all four extremities for three seconds. Squeeze buttocks together and pull stomach in.

all four extremities and the buttock muscles for three seconds (count of six). If you have any heart problem, do not tense all muscles at the same time. You will be more comfortable if you tense first the muscles of one arm, then those of the corresponding leg, now the other arm and the other leg. Tense buttock muscles separately. This way you do not overstrain yourself.

• Tense the muscles of your lower back region, then relax. Squeeze buttocks together, relax. Tense the shoulders, relax. Feet and ankles: tense, relax. Finally, hold the hands as stiff as possible, then relax.

Now the whole musculature has been warmed up a bit. Remember, at night the muscles are not called upon to work very much, and so they cool down. We warm them up to make them more flexible, either by taking a bath or by this brief isometric exercise.

• Lying on the bed on your back, retract your heels along the top of the bed toward your buttocks until the knees are all the way up. Now swing your arms all the way overhead and back until your thumbs touch the bed (fig. 6). Maintaining the same body position, rotate both arms inward and outward, so that palms point first up and then down. The reason for the posture—keeping your knees bent—is to keep the lower back flat. In this posture, we want to keep the stomach muscles contracted and avoid an upward curve (hollow) of the lower back, to avoid future back problems.

6. *With knees bent, swing arms overhead until thumbs touch bed.*

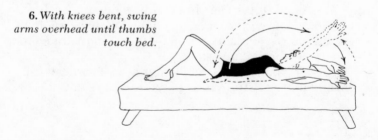

• Clasp your hands behind the back of your neck. Move elbows all the way out to press into the bed, and then move them upward until they touch (fig. 7).

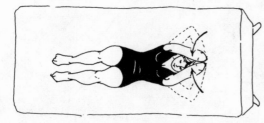

7. *Move elbows out to touch the bed. Then move elbows forward to touch one another. Hands are behind neck or behind head.*

• Extend both arms sideways, bend elbows, and try to touch the surface of the bed with your palms. Swing forearms up and touch the bed with back of your hands (fig. 8).

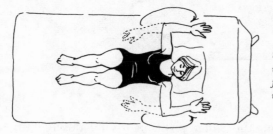

8. *Bend elbows to touch bed with palms. Then swing forearms up and touch bed with backs of hands.*

• With knees bent, raise your buttocks until the body forms a straight line (fig. 9). Lower the body to the bed.

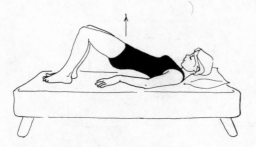

9. *With knees bent raise buttocks until body forms a straight line. Lower buttocks down again.*

• Sit up from the lying down position—if this is hard to do, use your elbows for support as you raise yourself up. Raise your knees and clasp your hands around them (fig. 10). Next, slowly lean back and hold the position for two to three seconds to exercise the abdominal muscles. Lower yourself down (fig. 11).

10. *Sit-ups*

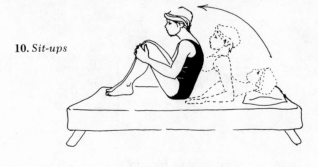

11. *Lean slowly backward and hold this position for two to three seconds.*

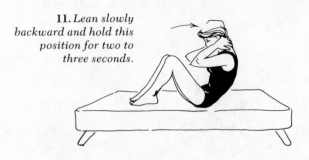

- Starting from the same position—lying down with knees up—do the following movements in sequence. Spread knees apart as far as they will go—do this slowly. If you feel tightness, contract the adductor muscles on the inside of thigh, relax and stretch farther out. Bring knees together again (fig. 12).

12. *Tense thighs, relax, then spread knees apart.*

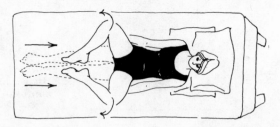

Clasp hands first around the lower part of your right thigh and bring it as close as possible to the chest (fig. 13). The left leg will tend to bend at the knee. Resist this by contracting all muscles of the thighs and buttocks for a few seconds; relax and then proceed to hold the left leg flat and down and the right leg drawn to the chest.

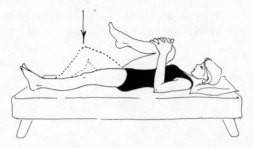

13. Push straight leg down, hold other knee to chest. Repeat with other leg.

• Next, clasp the hands around the right shinbone and pull the leg gently toward your chest (fig. 14). Careful—tight quadriceps muscles may produce pain in the knee. Don't go beyond the first feeling of pain.

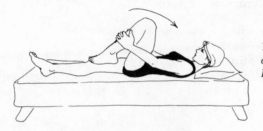

14. Pull shinbone toward chest. Stop short of pain. Repeat with other leg.

• Next, straighten the right leg and pull it gently up into the air by clasping the hands around the lower part of the thigh (fig. 15). Lower the right leg with the knee bent and dig the heel into the bed (fig. 16).

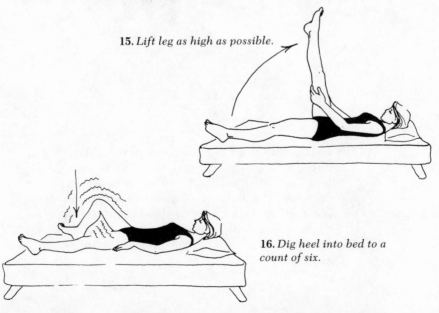

15. Lift leg as high as possible.

16. Dig heel into bed to a count of six.

Now lift leg up again with the aid of your hands and observe whether you get it up a little higher (fig. 17).

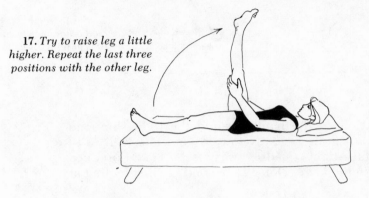

17. Try to raise leg a little higher. Repeat the last three positions with the other leg.

Complementary Exercise

Repeat this leg stretching with the other leg.

• Lie on the bed with legs flat and straight. Place your right heel above your left knee and lower your right knee as close as possible to the surface of the bed (fig. 18).

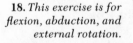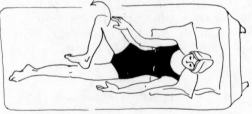

18. This exercise is for flexion, abduction, and external rotation.

Complementary Exercise

Repeat with the other leg.

• Lying with your legs straight and slightly spread, rotate the legs slowly inward as far as possible; your feet will form an angle of about forty-five degrees (fig. 19). Hold the position for one or two seconds. Next, rotate legs outward slowly and deliberately, all the way out. Hold position at the end of the range for one or two seconds. Repeat once, rotating once, back and forth.

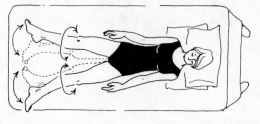

19. *Rotate leg slowly inward, all the way, then outward. Do this a few times.*

• Spread your legs apart as far as you can, moving slowly and deliberately, and dig heels in to provide resistance. If you are able to place your heels just beyond the edges of your bed (fig. 20), press both feet firmly against the edge of the bed. Keep legs firm at the knee. Tense leg muscle as if you were trying to bring the legs together. Hold contraction for two or three seconds, then relax and try to move legs farther apart.

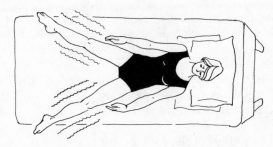

20. *Spread legs apart, strain as if to pull them together, spread them a little farther.*

• Roll over on your stomach and try to lift your shoulders and head off the surface of the bed once or twice (fig. 21). Lower head. Try to lift your legs, one at a time, off the bed. Then, if you can, lift both legs at the same time—slightly.

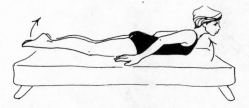

21. *Lift head and shoulders off bed once or twice, then try to lift legs a little.*

Next, flex your knees so that your heels approach your buttocks as closely as possible, to stretch the quadriceps muscles (fig. 22). To extend the range, tense the quadriceps muscles (muscle-setting), then flex the knees again. It is hard to become aware of whether you are extending your range unless someone tells you or unless you feel your heels touching your buttocks. You cannot do better than that.

22. *Swing legs toward buttocks. Tense thigh muscles, relax, try to come closer to buttocks.*

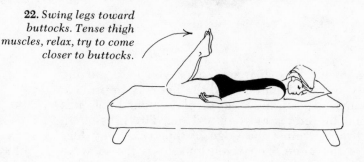

• Turn over again on your back and raise yourself to sit up, using your elbows as little as possible.

Remember to tense muscles and relax just prior to reaching for the end of a range in each motion. We have tensed all muscles of the four limbs at the beginning of the exercise. This gave us a general initial warm-up. However, as we practice an individual range we want to once more warm up the muscles around a particular joint.

• Sit at the edge of the bed with your feet on the floor. Lean back as far as you can, without supporting yourself with your hands or elbows, and swing back again (fig. 23). This is a good substitute exercise for strengthening very weak abdominal muscles; it is easier to do than the sit-up.

23. *Lean back as far as possible and swing up again to a straight sitting position. This is an easier substitute for the "lean back," fig. 11.*

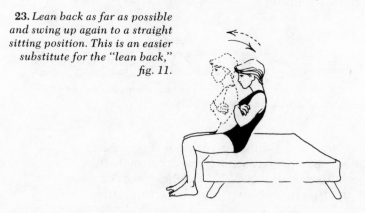

Daily Five-Minute Tense-Relax-and-Stretch Routine

Next, lean over to one side until you have to catch yourself by raising yourself with your hand (fig. 24). Sit up straight and lean to the other side.

• Do the motions here and in the next exercise while sitting on the edge of the bed or in a chair.

Bring one knee close to your chest with the hands clasped around the thigh. Touch your nose to the knee (fig. 25). Repeat for the other knee.

Raise one leg and tense the quadriceps muscle on top of your thigh for one or two seconds, as hard as possible (fig. 26). Repeat with the other leg.

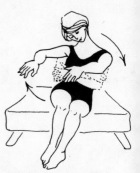

24. *Lean to one side until you must catch your balance by raising your arms. Then lean to the other side.*

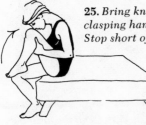

25. *Bring knee close to nose, clasping hands around thigh. Stop short of pain in the back.*

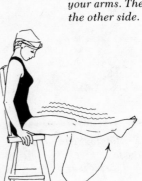

26. *Raise one leg at a time and tense the quadriceps a second or two as hard as possible.*

• With the heels on the ground, rotate both ankles so that the toes make a circle (fig. 27). Tense your toes, spread them apart, bring them together again, and curl. Relax.

• Go through all the ranges of motion of your neck. Move your head sideways toward your shoulder, first all the way to one side, then to the other (fig. 28). Don't forget to tense your neck muscles hard and relax before completing the ranges in all neck exercises.

27. *Circle each foot with heels on the floor. Also spread toes, curl toes.*

28. *Move the head sideways, first to one side then the other.*

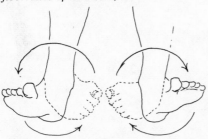

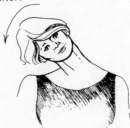

Rotate your head left and then right, all the way (fig. 29). Bend your head forward, touching your chin to your chest (fig. 30). Finally, bend it backward until the back of your head touches the nape of your neck (fig. 31). If you cannot reach this far, tense your neck muscles, as if to move in the opposite direction, relax, and try to move a little further down.

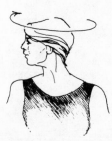

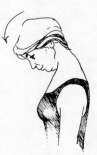

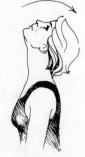

29. *Rotate the head all the way, first to the left and then the right.*

30. *Bend the head forward to touch chin to the chest.*

31. *Bend the head back until it touches the nape of the neck.*

• Move your shoulders up and down (shrugging motion) and rotate them forward and backward (figs. 32, 33).

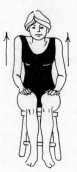

32. *Shrug your shoulders, move them up and down.*

33. *Rotate your shoulders forward and backward.*

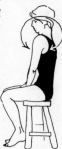

• Sit very straight with your shoulders drawn back. Hold for one or two seconds. It may help to tense the muscles that draw the shoulders inward, then relax and rotate shoulders all the way out and back (figs. 34, 35).

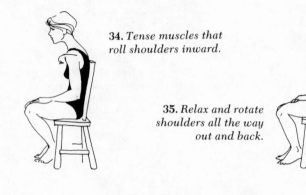

34. *Tense muscles that roll shoulders inward.*

35. *Relax and rotate shoulders all the way out and back.*

• Reach with your left hand over your shoulder to touch your left shoulder blade. At the same time reach with your right hand behind your back and try to meet your left hand (fig. 36). Next, reach with your right hand over your right shoulder and try to meet your left hand moving up behind the back (fig. 37).

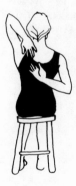
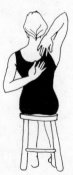

36. *Reach your left hand over your shoulder to touch your left shoulder blade. Simultaneously reach with your right hand behind your back to meet your left hand.*

37. *Reach the right hand over the right shoulder to meet the left hand moving up behind the back.*

• Spread your fingers far apart (fig. 38). Touch the tip of each finger to the base of the fingers with the fingertips, while holding the big knuckles straight (fig. 39). If you cannot perform this exercise while holding the big knuckles straight, exercise with the Hand Gym (fig. 40).

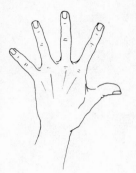

38. *Spread fingers as far apart as possible.*

39. *Curl fingers, trying to touch the base of each finger with the fingertip, while keeping the big knuckle (MCP joint) straight.*

40. *Curl fingers forcefully around foam rubber four times. Keep big knuckles "K" straight.*

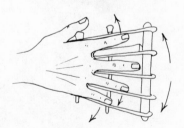

If you are using the Hand Gym, also spread the fingers apart against the walls, as strongly as possible, then bring them together again as strongly as possible against the walls (figs. 41a, b, c).

41a. *Spread fingers forcefully against the walls of the Gym for a count of six.*

41b. *Bring fingers together against the walls of the Gym forcefully for a count of six.*

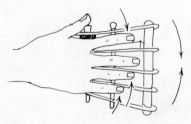

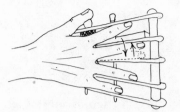

41c. *Press middle finger, first strongly, against one wall for a count of six, then against the opposite wall.*

• When you get up from your bed, make an effort to assume the best posture possible: stomach in, chest out, shoulders back, chin in, neck straight. Become aware of this posture so that you can assume it more and more often during the day. Remember, a good posture will permit you to breathe easier and will help to prevent back pain.

There you have twenty-three exercises, some of which are sequences for related sets of muscles. They take only five minutes to do once you are familiar with them. You need not necessarily do them in the sequence given here. You can use your own preferred sequence! And, as I said earlier, you can split the exercises, doing some of them while taking a bath or shower and some of them while lying down or sitting.

What is essential is that you (1) exercise every morning, and (2) try to reach the limit of each range conscientiously with slow, deliberate motions, with muscle tensing before the stretch, for highest efficiency.

This five-minute exercise routine accomplishes several things. It helps to maintain the strength of one of the most important muscles of the body—the quadriceps. In addition, the allover stretching makes you aware of your body and allows you to check your muscles and ranges to see if you are maintaining your ranges or whether there is any joint that is becoming more limited in its range. If this should be the case, consider carefully what you can do to treat this. Make a mental note to exercise this joint with special care on the evening of the week when you exercise that part of the body.

In the beginning of the book I suggested a nightly sequence of exercises. I repeat it here:

Monday night:	neck and jaw
Tuesday night:	shoulders and elbows
Wednesday night:	hands and wrists
Thursday night:	posture and upper back
Friday night:	lower back, hips, and knees
Saturday night:	feet and ankles

COUNTERING PAIN

☐ You may want to protect any particular joint that seems to be losing range, by keeping it warm. For the neck you may want to use a scarf; for the shoulders, a woollen undergarment or wool sweater; for the elbows, a sleeve-type small knee-warmer; for the wrists, a lightly wrapped Ace bandage; for your lower back and hips, a kidney (hip) warmer or woollen girdle (imported from Germany under the trade name Medima (fig. 42); for the knees, knee warmers; for the ankles, Ace bandages.*

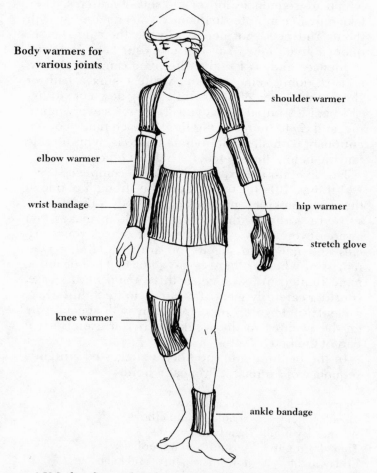

Body warmers for
various joints

shoulder warmer

elbow warmer

wrist bandage

hip warmer

stretch glove

knee warmer

ankle bandage

* U.S. distributor of Medima: Surgical Appliance Industries, 3960 Rosalyn Drive, Cincinnati, Ohio 45209

If a joint reacts with pain to the five-minute workout, it may be eased by hot compresses or, for hands and feet, a hot whirlpool bath. Ease a swollen finger joint by wearing a hand-rest splint, not only at night but perhaps also during part of the day. You may want to use stretch gloves during the night. These are known to help unswell fingers.

REMEMBER THE REWARDS

☐ In all these endeavors you do not consider yourself a patient, but a person committed to improving her or his body. You are doing the equivalent of Yoga or calisthenics to improve flexibility and strength and to maintain an elegant posture.

By now you will have learned just how far you can stretch your joints without doing them damage. If we live "within our joints," we can still enjoy many years of near-normal activity. We do not want to be hemmed in, to have to rest most of the time, but rather we want to be active. Minor muscular or ligamentous aches are inevitable. These we attend to quickly so that they are not aggravated, but are cured if possible.

A WORD TO CHRONIC ARTHRITICS

☐ As I said earlier, these exercises are not for those patients in the chronic phase of the disease, where joint destruction is quite evident, and where the disease activity remains high in spite of gold treatment or other medications. For such patients, even gentle exercises may place too much strain on the system and produce flare-ups. They have to exercise under close supervision of their physicians or therapists. Their hope must also be based on the promise offered by such procedures as synovectomies (removal of the inflamed synovium, the internal joint membrane), and surgical replacement of joints.

Those who so far have been spared such disability will, I hope, do the exercises with enthusiasm, optimism, and a firm purpose, to prevent unnecessary loss of function.

Directory of Aids

□ Exercise and self-help aids are listed in:

• *Home Health Care Catalogue* of Sears, Roebuck and Company, available free at Sears catalogue counters or by mail from Sears, Roebuck and Company, North Philadelphia, Pennsylvania 19132.
• *Catalogue* of Maddak Incorporated, available free by mail from Maddak Inc., Pequannock, New Jersey 07440. Maddak products are available directly by mail or from selected surgical and medical supply stores which carry their products.

The next two excellent publications list hundreds of self-help devices and sources.

• *Self-Help Manual for Arthritic Patients,* published by The Arthritis Foundation, $3.00, from your local Arthritis Foundation chapter or by mail from Arthritis Foundation National Headquarters, 3400 Peachtree Road North East, Atlanta, Georgia 30326.
• *Mealtime Manual for People with Disabilities and the Aging,* $3.50, from Campbell Soup Company, Box MM 56, Camden, New Jersey 08101.

CHAPTER FOUR

Aids for Applying Heat

ELECTRIC HOT PAD, THERMOPHORE.   Supplies faster and more heat than normal heating pads, available in surgical supply stores, $50.00.

WHIRLPOOL ATTACHMENT FOR A BATHTUB. $80.00-$300.00, Sears, Roebuck. The jet can easily be directed at feet and legs, and, with a special attachment, at neck, back, and shoulders.

MASSAGE SHOWER HEADS.   Approximately $15.00 for the overhead shower and $30.00 for the hand-held shower, at Sears, Roebuck, drugstores, and department stores. Overhead unit suitable for neck, shoulders, and back. Hand-held units suitable for hips and knees.

A COMPACT SELF-CONTAINED WHIRLPOOL.   Available from Sears, Roebuck catalogue, 8AH2262, $29.88, see figure 63, page 142. It is useful for feet, hands, and elbows.

BODY WARMERS.   For knees, hips, elbows, hands, and feet, made of angora wool and elastic fibers, are especially useful for the arthritic. Medima Angora Warmers, made in Germany, are distributed in the United States by Surgical Appliance Industries, 3960 Rosalyn Drive, Cincinnati, Ohio 45209.

KNEE WARMERS.   Also available from Dr. Scholl and department stores, at approximately $5.00.

ELASTIC BANDAGES (SUCH AS THE ACE BANDAGE). Available at most drugstores. The 3½-inch width is useful for the ankle, knee, and wrist because it keeps these joints warm and stabilized.

CHAPTER SIX

Aids and Exercise Equipment for the Neck

CERVICAL PILLOWS.   Available at surgical supply stores for approximately $9.00. If not satisfactory try to make one yourself as shown in figure 28, page 112.

HEAD TRACTION SET TO RELIEVE NECK PAIN.   Available for $12.50 through surgical supply stores or rehabilitation equipment stores. Doctor's supervision required.

CHAPTER SEVEN

Exercise Equipment for Shoulders and Elbows

HORIZONTAL GYM BAR.   For mounting in doorway, Maddak catalog H70960, $16.20, also available from sports and department stores.

INFLATABLE BEACH BALL.   Preferred size 38 inches (1 m) circumference, also usable for exercising hips.

6-INCH- (15 CM) WIDE DENTAL DAM (THIN RUBBER). Try to obtain a length of at least 88 inches (2.26 m) through your dentist or a dental supply company. (A rubberized belt or even a leather belt may be used.) Also usable for exercising hips.

WEIGHTS.   For one pound use a box of salt. Two-pound ankle weights from Maddak, catalogue H70970, $15.00 pr. Three pounds, H70971, $17.25 pr., is usable for exercising knees.

AN OVER-THE-DOOR PULLEY.   Available for $16.50 at surgical supply or rehabilitation stores. A simple pulley can be made by yourself: see figure 32, page 131.

CHAPTER EIGHT

Aids and Exercise Equipment for Hands

THE HAND GYM.   Maddak catalogue F70900, $20.00, Sears, Roebuck catalogue 8AH1353, $18.95.

HAND REST SPLINT.   Figure 15a, page 153 can be made to order by an occupational therapist, as prescribed by a physician.

SWAN-NECK RING.   Figure 16a, page 155 can be made up by an orthotics department, as prescribed by a physician.

THUMB SPLINT.   Can be prescribed by your physician to help extend the MCP joint of the thumb, while keeping the CM joint (carpal metacarpal) at the base of thumb movable. This small splint can be stabilized with Velcro around your wrist. You may have to search for an orthotics or an occupational therapy department willing to make it.

OVERSIZED KEY HOLDER.   Reduces strength necessary to open your door. Maddak catalogue H75412, $4.50; and Sears, Roebuck catalogue 8AH1373, $3.69.

A PRACTICAL JAR OPENER.   Saves your knuckles. Maddak catalogue F75346, $5.25; Sears, Roebuck catalogue 8AH1366, $4.99.

STRETCH GLOVES.   Isotoner Gloves, price range $10.00–15.00. Therapeutic stretch gloves are also available from surgical supply or rehabilitation stores and selected drugstores under the name of Futura, at $20.00. Stretch gloves are especially useful for comfort at night.

RUBBER CAPS.   Slip over doorknobs. Available through surgical supply stores, at about $3.00.

CHAPTER TEN

Aids and Exercise Equipment for Hips and Knees

INFLATABLE BEACH BALL.   Preferred size 38 inches (1 m) circumference, also usable for exercising shoulders and elbows.

6-INCH- (15 CM) WIDE DENTAL DAM (THIN RUBBER). Try to obtain a length of at least 88 inches (2.26 m) through your dentist or a dental supply company. (A rubberized belt or even a leather belt may be used). Also usable for exercising shoulders and elbows.

WEIGHTS.   For one pound use a box of salt. Two-pound ankle weights from Maddak, catalogue H70970, $15.00 pr. Three pounds, H70971, $17.25 pr., is usable for exercising shoulders and elbows.

HIGH SEAT CUSHIONS.   Take stress off knees and hips and make sitting down and rising from chairs more comfortable. Maddak catalogue H76665, 4 inches (10 cm), $19.95; H76666, 6 inches (15 cm), $24.45; see figure 81, page 233.

ELEVATED TOILET SEATS.   Maddak catalogue F72580, 4-inch (10 cm), $18.00. Sears, Roebuck elevated adjustable toilet seat from 3 to 6 inches, catalogue 8AH1175, $15.95; Maddak catalogue F72586, 6-inch (15 cm), $25.00.

A VARIETY OF REACHING AIDS.   Available from Maddak for $7.50 to $43.50, page 51 of their catalogue 479. Sears, Roebuck sells a trigger-controlled extension grip to extend your reach, catalogue 8AH1370, $14.89.

LONG SHOEHORN.   Can be very useful. Maddak catalogue H73823, 23-inch (60 cm), $7.80; 73824, 17½-inch (44 cm), $2.00.

A SMALL UTILITY CART OR TEA WAGON.   If both hands are occupied with cane or crutches I find it convenient to move objects on this item. Available from Sears, Roebuck at $17.00 and up. Catalogue 11G7097C.

Sock aid.   Permits you to pull sock on and off without bending. Maddak catalogue F73841, $6.15. Sears, Roebuck catalogue 8AH1377, $5.89.

Elastic shoelaces.   Permit shoes to be slipped on and off without tying or untying. Maddak catalogue F73814, black, $3.95, 3 pr.

Canes, crutches, walkers, wheelchairs.   Described in catalogues, but are best fitted by your therapist on prescription of a physician.

Exercise bicycle.   An excellent muscle and endurance trainer, nearly as good as a regular bicycle. Check with your physician if you should use one. A variety is shown in the Sears, Roebuck *Home Health Catalogue.* They are often also available locally, and can also be rented from surgical supply stores.

CHAPTER ELEVEN

Foot Aids

Metatarsal Pad.   Available in various sizes from Dr. Scholl at approximately $1.00 pr. Select the proper size according to men's/women's shoe size. Insert in shoe, directly behind the arch. See figure 6, page 241.

Toe dividers.   Available from Dr. Scholl. The one between the big toe and the next toe is especially useful to prevent the big toe from turning in. See figure 5, page 240.

Arch supports.   To support the longitudinal arch as well as the metatarsal arch. They are usually custom prescribed by a physician. Standardized arch supports are available from Dr. Scholl for various shoe sizes. They cost only a small fraction of the individualized fitted ones, but check them for comfort.

Bibliography

1. GENERAL BOOKS ON ARTHRITIS

☐ Bland, J. H. *Arthritis: Medical Treatment and Home Care.* New York: Collier Books, 1962.

☐ Blau, S. P., and Schultz, D. *Arthritis.* Garden City, N.Y.: Doubleday, 1974.

☐ Casley-Smith, J. R. "How the Lymphatic System Works." *Lymphology,* 1 (1968): 77–80.

☐ Corrigan, A. B. *Living with Arthritis.* New York: Grosset and Dunlap, 1971.

☐ Cousins, Norman. *The Anatomy of an Illness.* New York: Norton & Co., 1979.

☐ Crain, Darrell C. *The Arthritis Handbook: A Patient's Manual on Arthritis, Rheumatism, and Gout.* 2d rev. ed. Jericho, N.Y.: Exposition Press, 1972.

☐ Decker, John L. "From Willow Bark to Cytotoxies, The Management of Rheumatoid Arthritis." *Medical Times* 105 (November, 1977): 28–34.

☐ Ekblom, B.; Lovgren, O.; Alderin, M.; Fridstrom, M.; and Satterstrom, G. "Effect of short-term physical training on patients with rheumatoid Arthritis II." *Scandinavian Journal of Rheumatology* 4 (1975): 87.

☐ Fries, James F., M.D. *Arthritis. A Comprehensive Guide.* Reading, Mass.: Addison-Wesley, 1979.

☐ Healey, Louis A. *Long-Term Management of Rheumatoid Arthritis: Going Beyond the Relief of Pain.* The Upjohn Co., 1978.

☐ Healey, Louis A.; Wilske, Kenneth R.; and Hansen, Bob H. *Beyond the Copper Bracelet: What You Should Know About Arthritis.* 2d. ed. Bowie, Md.: Charles Press, 1977.

☐ Hollander, Joseph Lee, ed. *Arthritis and Allied Conditions, A Textbook of Rheumatology.* 7th ed. Philadelphia: Lea & Febiger, 1966.

☐ Johnson, G. Timothy. *Coping With Arthritis.* New York: Newspaperbooks, 1977.

☐ Keeton, William T. *Biological Science.* Toronto: George J. McLeod, 1967.

☐ Kitay, William. *Understanding Arthritis.* New York: Monarch Press, 1977.

☐ Lamont-Havers, Ronald W., and Hislop, Helen J., eds. *Arthritis and Related Disorders.* New York: American Physical Therapy Association, 1965.

☐ Machover, S., and Sapecky, A. J. "Effect of Isometric Exercises on the Quadriceps Muscle in Patients with Rheumatoid Arthritis." *Archives of Physical Medicine* 47 (November, 1966): 737.

☐ The Professional Manual Subcommittee of the Education Committee, Allied Health Professions Section of The Arthritis Foundation. *Arthritis Manual for Allied Health Professionals.* New York: The Arthritis Foundation, 1973.

☐ Resnick, Donald, M.D. "Arthrography in the Evaluation of Arthritic Disorders of the Wrist." *Radiology* 113 (November, 1974): 331–340.

☐ Rusznyak, I.; Foldi, M.; and Szabo, G. *Lymphatics and Lymph Circulation.* London: Pergamon Press, 1960.

☐ Swezey, Robert L. *Arthritis: Rational Therapy and Rehabilitation.* Philadelphia & London: W. B. Saunders, 1978.

☐ Winocur, William. "A Client Looks at Caring For the Arthritis Patient." *Arthritis Newsletter* 13: no. 2, pp. 1–4.

2. JOINTS AND JOINT PROTECTION

☐ Beetham, William P.; Polley, Howard F.; Slocumb, Charles H.; and Weaver, Walt F. *Physical Examination of the Joints.* Philadelphia & London: W. B. Saunders, 1965.

☐ Brattstrom, Merete. *Principles of Joint Protection in Chronic Rheumatic Disease.* Chicago: Year Book Medical Publishers, 1975.

☐ Daniels, Lucille; Williams, Marian; and Worthingham, Catherine. *Muscle Testing Technique of Manual Examination.* 2d ed. Philadelphia & London: W. B. Saunders, 1956.

☐ Fox, Theodore A., ed. *Manual of Orthopaedic Surgery.* Chicago: American Orthopaedic Association, 1966.

☐ Kapandji, I. A. *The Physiology of the Joints.* Vol. 1, *Upper Limb.* Vol. 2, *Lower Limb.* Edinburgh, London, New York: Churchill Livingstone, 1970.

☐ Klinger, Judith Lannefeld, for Allied Health Professions Section of The Arthritis Foundation. *Self-Help Manual for Arthritis Patients.* New York: The Arthritis Foundation, 1974.

3. EXERCISES

☐ The Arthritis Foundation. *Home Care Programs in Arthritis, A Manual for Patients.* New York: The Arthritis Foundation, 1969.

☐ Fallon, Michael, and Saunders, Jim. *Muscle Building For Beginners.* New York: Arc Books, 1964.

☐ Fellman, N., and Hinlopen-Bonrath, E. *Bewwgungsubungen fur Rheumakranke.* Zurich: Schweizerische Rheumaliga, 1974.

☐ Hettinger, Theodor. *Fit sein–fit bleiben: Isometrisches Muskeltraining fur den Alltag.* Stuttgart, Georg Thieme Verlag, 1977.

☐ ——*Isometrisches Muskeltraining.* 4th ed. Stuttgart: Georg Thieme Verlag, 1972.

☐ Jensen, H. P. *Bewugungsubungen fur die Wirbelsaule.* Hanover: Efeka Friedrich & Kaufman Arzeneimittelfabrik, n.d.

☐ Kaganas, G. Die häusliche Pflege des Rheumakranken. Zurich: Schweizerischen Rheumaliga, n.d.

☐ Klein-Vogelbach, Susanne. *Therapeutische Ubungen zur funktionellen Bewugungslehre, Analysen und Rezepte.* Berlin, Heidelberg & New York: Springer-Verlag; and Heidelberg: Stiftunge Rehabilitation, 1978.

☐ Knott, Margaret, and Voss, Dorothy E. *Proprioceptive Neuromuscular Facilitation, Patterns and Techniques.* 2d ed. New York: Harper & Row, 1968.

☐ The Mason Clinic. *Therapeutic Program for the Patient with Arthritis.* 2d ed. Seattle: The Mason Clinic, n.d.

☐ Mensendieck, Bess, M.D. *Look Better, Feel Better.* New York: Harper & Row, 1954.

☐ Morehouse, Laurence E., and Miller, Augustus T. *Physiology of Exercise.* 6th ed. Saint Louis: C. V. Mosby, 1971.

☐ Morehouse, Laurence E., and Gross, Leonard. *Total Fitness in 30 Minutes a Week*. New York: Simon and Schuster, 1975.

☐ Mossfeldt, Folke, and Miller, Mary Susan. *SAS In-the-Chair Exercise Book*. New York: Bantam Books, 1979.

☐ Müller, Erich A. "Influence of Training and of Inactivity on Muscle Strength." *Archives of Physical Medicine and Rehabilitation* (August, 1970): 449–62.

☐ The President's Council on Physical Fitness, Sports, and the Administration on Aging. *The Fitness Challenge . . . in the Later Years, an exercise program for older Americans*. DHEW Publication (SRS) 72-20802. Washington: Department of Health, Education, and Welfare, 1968, 1972 reprint.

☐ *Royal Canadian Air Force Exercise Plans for Physical Fitness*. New York: Pocket Books, 1972.

☐ Scharll, Martha. *Aktiv im Alter durch Gymnastik*. Stuttgart: Georg Thieme Verlag, 1976.

☐ Spreads, Carola H. *Breathing, The ABCs*. New York: Harper & Row, 1978.

4. HAND EXERCISES

☐ Bens, Doris E., and Krewer, Semyon E. "The Hand Gym: An Exercise Apparatus for the Patient with Rheumatoid Arthritis." *Archives of Physical Medicine and Rehabilitation* 55 (October, 1974): 477–80.

☐ Cailliet, Rene. *Hand Pain and Impairment*. Philadelphia: F. A. Davis, 1971.

☐ Flatt, A. *The Care of the Rheumatoid Hand*. St. Louis: C. V. Mosby, 1963.

☐ Krewer, Semyon E. "Calibrated Grasping Tubes for Intrinsic-Plus Testing of Arthritic Hands." *Archives of Physical Medicine and Rehabilitation* 59 (June, 1978): 293–94.

☐ Schaufler, Judith; Sverdlik, Samuel S.; Baker, Anita; and Krewer, Semyon E. " 'Hand Gym' for Patients with Arthritic Hand Disabilities: Preliminary Report." *Archives of Physical Medicine and Rehabilitation* 59 (May, 1978): 221–26.

☐ Wynn-Parry, C. B. *Rehabilitation of the Hand*. London: Buttersworth, 1973.

☐ Zancolli, Eduardo. *Structural and Dynamic Bases of Hand Surgery*. Philadelphia: Lippincott, 1968.

5. DANCE AND YOGA

☐ Brown, Margaret C., Ed.D. *Movement Education: Its evolution and a modern approach*. Reading, Mass.: Addison-Wesley, 1969.

☐ Department of Tourism, Ministry of Transport and Communications, Government of India. *The Dance in India.* Calcutta: Sree Saraswatty Press, 1964.

☐ Gelabert, Raoul: as told to Como, William. *Raoul Gelabert's Anatomy for the Dancer, with Exercises to Improve Technique and Prevent Injuries.* Vol. 1. New York: Danad, 1964. Vol. 2, 1964.

☐ Lipson. Goldie, *Rejuvenation Through Yoga.* New York: Pyramid Books, 1963.

☐ Pearlman, Barbara. *Barbara Pearlman's Dance Exercises.* Garden City, N.Y.: Dolphin Books, Doubleday, 1977.

☐ Rama, Swami; Ballentine, Rudolph, M.D.; and Hymes, Alan, M.D. *Science of Breath.* Honesdale, Pa.: The Himalayan International Institute of Yoga Science and Philosophy, 1979.

☐ Vishnudevananda, Swami. *The Complete Illustrated Book of Yoga.* New York: Pocket Books, 1960.

6. BACK EXERCISES

☐ Kraus, Hans. *Backache, Stress, and Tension.* New York: Pocket Books, 1969.

☐ Lettvin, Maggie. *Maggie's Back Book, Healing the Hurt in Your Lower Back.* Boston: Houghton Mifflin, 1976.

☐ Root, Leon, and Kiernan, Thomas. *Oh, My Aching Back.* New York: Signet, New American Library, 1975.

☐ Wayne, Jerry. *The Bad Back Book.* New York: Dell, 1974.

7. PAIN AND EXERCISE

☐ Cailliet, Rene. *Foot and Ankle Pain.* Philadelphia: F. A. Davis, 1968.

☐ ——*Knee Pain and Disability.* Philadelphia: F. A. Davis, 1973.

☐ ——*Neck and Arm Pain.* Philadelphia: F. A. Davis, 1964.

☐ ——*Soft Tissue Pain and Disability.* Philadelphia: F. A. Davis, 1977.

☐ Jacobsen, Edward, M.D. *Progressive Relaxation.* Chicago: University of Chicago Press, 1938.

☐ Marbach, Joseph J., D.D.S. "Arthritis of the Temporomandibular Joints and Facial Pain." *Bulletin on the Rheumatic Diseases* 27: no. 8, pp. 918–21.

Index

285